A memoir of love and loss

A Journey of Love
a dementia caregiver's story

Rosemarie Jordan

© 2024 by Rosemarie Jordan

ISBN: 979-8-9905354-8-0 (ppb)

Printed in the United States of America

All rights reserved. No part of this publication may be reproduced, distributed, or transmitted in any form or by any means, including photocopying, recording, or other electronic or mechanical methods, without prior written permission of the publisher, except as permitted by U.S. copyright law.

For privacy reasons, some names, locations, and dates may have been changed.

All reader comments are welcome. I'd love to hear from you at:
adementiacaregiverstory@yahoo.com

PRAISE FOR
A Journey of Love
a dementia caregiver's story

"Rosemarie shared her own raw, moving, and profoundly real account of the challenges, sacrifices, and poignant moments of connection individuals with dementia and their caregivers experience as they traverse the dementia journey. She emerges as a powerful voice of advocacy. Through her personal story, she sheds light on the silent struggles of caregivers, illuminating the urgent need for a broader conversation around dementia care. A Journey of Love is not just another book, but a badly needed catalyst for change when it comes to standard of care for those with dementia and increased support for the family caregivers who love them."

Martina Rutledge, caregiver
Portland, Oregon

"A Journey of Love was written directly from the heart. I admire Rosemarie for bearing her heart and soul and sharing a part of her life, so others can get a glimpse of what caregivers go through caring for their loved ones. All caregivers will be able to relate to some part of this book, whether their loved ones are at the beginning or the later stages of the disease. We have all been through some part of it."

Wylene Wiechmann, caregiver
Mesa, Arizona

"This book is amazing. I absolutely fell in love with Gary and Rose! As a caregiver myself, I identified similar situations/moments in my journey. The advice and resources at the back of the book are priceless pieces of information to someone just starting this journey. Caregiving is a gift from the heart and is not for everyone, it is even more so with a dementia/Alzheimer's patient. The angels that are found along the way are true blessings. Rose has inspired me to do more for others on this journey."

Jana Votava, caregiver
Garvin, MN

"Heartbreaking and brutally honest. This poignant walk through the journey of dementia caregiving and unconditional love of another soul is a must read for everyone. This is a candid illustration of the devastation a diagnosis brings, and the compassion that lives in the depths of our souls."

Melinda Tapanes, hospice volunteer
Whittier, NC

Dedication and in honor of:
Gary

*The best friend and lover a girl could have.
I did it, babe!*

"And once the storm is over, you won't remember how you made it through, how you managed to survive. You won't even be sure, in fact, whether the storm is really over. But one thing is certain. When you come out of the storm, you won't be the same person who walked in. That's what this storm's all about."

HARUKI MURAKAMI
Kafka on the Shore

Author's Note

Writing about the most painful period of my life was more difficult than I imagined. I tried to find the good parts of the journey. There were moments that Gary and I would laugh together and share the friendship that created a bond so strong even dementia could not destroy it. Dementia never stole Gary's heart. His heart knew me and others until he took his last breath.

Initially, most dementia caregivers do not have all the facts about the disease. They do not know how it will affect them, financially, mentally, or physically. They do not know the time it involves, how ugly the disease gets, how isolated they will be, or the mental imprisonment of dementia. They do not think that some family members will disappear and will not call, visit, offer respite, help, or support. Their primary reason for assuming the care of their loved one is love. Without that love, there would be no caregiver journey. Hence the title of my book, "A Journey of Love." Love is what propels most dementia caregivers to accept the responsibility of care. Their reward is knowing they are helping another human being.

I hope this book validates some of the emotions, heartaches, and exhaustion many caregivers experience. So often we feel no one is listening and we are alone on this journey. At times I feared I would not make it to the other side. When I began to put excerpts from my writing on dementia support groups, I got over 2,000 hits and dozens of requests from caregivers to be their voice. I hope this book does justice to our selfless acts of compassion and love for our loved ones.

For the millions of dementia warriors who do the impossible every day caring for loved ones with dementia singlehandedly, you have my utmost respect. Taking care of someone and expecting nothing in return is an incredibly unselfish act that demonstrates the best of humanity. Our dementia journeys as caregivers, although different, are alike in many ways. Abandonment, anticipatory grief, physical and emotional exhaustion, aloneness, and isolation are common themes. I did my best to explore each one.

Dementia is vastly different for every individual. Gary did not suffer from hallucinations, paranoia, or refusing to eat or drink, and he did not spend his days screaming or slamming doors, etc. These challenges make the journey more difficult. Gary also had long-term insurance providing me with access to a facility and respite. Many fellow warriors do not have that opportunity because they lack long-term insurance, and the cost of care is exorbitant. I was blessed to be able to provide Gary with additional love and support from these facilities. The staff became my extended family.

For those reading this book who are not caregivers, I hope you have the courage to read the entire book. It will make you knowledgeable of what millions of dementia caregivers experience during the journey. Before I walked the walk, I was ignorant of this disease. Someone said to me, "I may not be on your journey, but I know what dementia is." Reading a description of a disease is not the same as experiencing it. This book will give you an opportunity to step into the shoes of at least one dementia warrior. There are nearly seven million of us, and the numbers keep growing.

Hopefully people will be encouraged and help caregivers by providing love, support, and respite. Dementia care needs a wider audience. There are not nearly enough resources for caregivers.

I intend on using proceeds from this book to help dementia caregivers. I currently provide funds to caregivers for massages, haircuts, manicures, pedicures, etc., through an agency respite grant program. If you have an idea where proceeds can be directed, I'd love to hear from you.

Feel free to reach out to me at adementiacaregiverstory@yahoo.com.

God Bless

Prelude

The Wink

October 2023

No matter how many visits I made, I still woke up enveloped in sadness. Being on this journey for ten years did not soften the effects of seeing Gary's decline. One part of me wanted to go, the other part begged me not to. My heart always won. It pushed me forward.

I usually found Gary in the lunchroom with his wheelchair pushed close to the table. I'd give him a once over, noting any changes.

"Hi, sweetheart. Hang on," I'd say. "I'll be right back."

"Okay," he'd reply.

I'd go across the room and grab a terry bib. After securing it around his neck, I'd cut up his meal. The food quality was an improvement on the last facility. I pushed a caramel frappe toward him that I had purchased earlier. Gary still enjoyed his coffee drinks.

He reached for it. "Thanks," he replied with a half-smile. Dementia had not stolen his gratitude.

I settled in and observed him eating. Today his coordination was good, and he was able to get the fork to his mouth. I decided to assist the man at the other side of the table.

I froze my emotions as I felt the suffering in the room. I did this throughout the journey. I turned my feelings into ice cubes that refused to melt into tears. I did not want Gary to see my sadness. He'd be unhappy if he saw me cry.

Some dementia patients roamed the room, and others sat around dining tables, still able to feed themselves. And then there were those like Gary, who had lost their mobility and were in wheelchairs. They often needed assistance with feeding. A few aides saw me from across the room and waved. The aide that usually welcomed me with a hug was not there. I saw no other visitors in the room.

I steeled myself to concentrate on Gary, although it was a struggle for me. My mind and body were saturated with the surroundings. I searched the tables for the assisted living residents, as they were more able in mind and body. The sense of hopelessness for those in end-stage dementia trapped my mind between life and death. I felt encased in a seatbelt and wanted to wiggle free to join the other residents at their table.

I felt disbelief that this was my new reality. It felt surreal. A part of life I never thought I'd visit. Let alone live. And certainly not with Gary, who was always a healthy man.

I looked over at him. I didn't want him to feel or see my pain. But my face showed everything.

And then it happened.

He winked at me. And then that familiar smirk from forty years ago when we dated. Gary was oblivious to his good looks, with his jet-black hair and blue eyes. When we were separated in a room, I'd search for his presence. When my eyes found him, he'd wink at me and smirk as if to say, "Hey there, beautiful." I'd always smile back with a happy thought that he was mine.

No, it can't be. *I imagined that.*

And then he did it again. First the wink. Then the welcoming smirk that extended to the corner of his blue eyes.

It whispered to me. "I'm still here. It's gonna be okay, my beautiful wife."

I smiled back reassuringly, willing myself not to cry.

What is wrong with my husband?

"We should not confuse information with knowledge."

T. S. ELIOT

2011

Gary and I bought a home in 2006 on the North Carolina coast without selling our mountain home in western North Carolina. The real estate market was hot, and a bank appraisal predicted a significant growth in profit. Although the risk existed that our mountain home would not sell, it appeared minimal and worth taking. I was ready to return to a more citified life.

Who could foresee that within a year the nation would enter a housing crisis. In life, some things, like the real estate market and dementia, are impossible to predict. Despite our careful planning, life has a way of forcing us to change course. But we march forward and do the best we can with the cards that have been dealt.

After five years of suffering under two mortgages, electric bills, heating bills, property taxes, and maintenance on two homes, the financial stress was unbearable. I managed the checkbook, so I alone had the burden of knowing what this was doing to our assets. Gary had no interest in our finances or managing them.

I began to force a decision to short sell the coastal home, which had less equity. I laid out a ledger detailing our finances over the last five years. The debt, the mortgage payments, the hit our stocks had taken, the loss of my most recent job, and the $12,000 spent on a new well at our mountain home.

Gary sat stoically on the couch. No amount of prompting for a solution to fix this problem elicited any response. He sat staring straight ahead. His apathy was downright infuriating.

"Say something," I demanded. "Anything, anything at all! Give me a hint. What the hell should we do?"

No response. And then in a whisper, "What do you want me to do?" This was so uncharacteristic of Gary, who in the past would offer a solution prompting a discussion on the best course of action.

In the months following, I noticed Gary had no interest in any activities. In previous years, we always enjoyed an annual blueberry festival. We looked forward to all the blueberry treats that the community made. However, that year Gary walked through the fair downcast, looking bored and unhappy. Even the enthusiasm he once had for home projects or going on trips was nonexistent. I began feeling disconnected from the man I said vows with in 1986. I felt emotionally neglected and very lonely.

Initially I thought the mood change was his age. He was twelve years older than I. Perhaps he was having a midlife crisis, or he was losing interest in me. Maybe the stress and weariness of supporting two homes was wearing on him. On days I was honest with myself, I admitted that our marriage had been struggling for years. But now his apathy was exacerbating the struggle to the point that I no longer knew my friend and partner.

In December I asked him for a separation. "Okay, if that's what you want," he replied. With raised eyebrows I stared at him with disbelief. He offered nothing else, not even an argument. The husband that I remembered would have fought to keep me. He'd share how much he loved me and tell me that leaving him would cause a hole in his heart. He'd ask, "What can I do so that you won't leave? Just tell me, and I'll do it. I love you!" What was causing this change in attitude? This apathetic mood? His inability to focus on decisions that needed to be made?

2012

In a marriage nearly everything is done in partnership. When you disconnect from someone after many years, it's like a limb is missing. Or a persistent nag, like when you forget to put on the wristwatch that's graced your arm for years. Nothing feels quite the same. Being separated was more difficult than I thought. And dealing with questions from relatives and friends added to the discomfort.

"Did he cheat?" No.
"Did he lie?" No.
"Did he try to control your life?" No.
"Did he deny you independence to do what you wanted?" No.

Few understood why I wanted out of our marriage. When I shared that I felt I was the only adult in the house it did not elicit any empathy. When I explained he was not the same as the man I married, they'd look at me perplexed. "Surely you jest. What man is?" I needed to sit with that thought for a while. Are other marriages like that? Do partners change that much? Gary and I started our relationship as best friends. I felt lonelier living with this stranger than I would by myself.

I wanted someone to take part in my life and enjoy laughter and quiet late-night talks. I needed my husband to share in important decisions that needed to be made. I simply longed for the man I had married twenty-six years before.

But I had felt like I was living on an island bathed only by my tears the last five years. The management of our lives, investments, finances, and other responsibilities that I had easily assumed years before were so much more challenging with two homes. Carrying this additional burden was causing me an increased amount of stress. Coupled with a forty plus–hour work week and Gary's recent change of attitude, my life felt unbearable.

I loved this man. I tried to talk. I tried to ignore it. I tried to focus on counting my blessings. I tried to convince myself that the things

I craved and wanted weren't important. The gnawing for something more in a relationship persisted.

When Gary appeared lost in his own world without a compass, I remembered that he always was a little daffy. A little slow to the take. As an example, when we were dating, he promised to pick up chicken and be right over. Within twenty minutes he was knocking on my door.

"Where's the chicken?" I asked.

It was then that he realized he had put it on the roof of his car while navigating his keys and driven off without it.

There was also the time we went to the beach with his son from an earlier marriage. We laid our blanket down and got our towels out. His son and I watched him run down to the water wearing only his underwear. Gary had removed his shorts, forgetting he had no swim trucks underneath. His son and I were bent over in laughter screaming, "Come back, you're in your underwear!"

So, when his moods and lack of focus began, it did not set off alarms. I didn't consider anything other than Gary's age, personality, stress level, or traits his character always wore.

I asked Gary to return to our mountain home. It had been abandoned for six years, and it needed repairs before it would be marketable. I decided to stay in our coastal home and get it ready for sale. The time apart would give us time to think and process how we wanted to proceed.

Once he left, I found him communicating less and less and withdrawing more and more from our relationship. This was also not the response from Gary that I'd expect. The Gary I knew would not desert or give up on his best friend. He would call daily to check on me, engage in conversation, and tell me what he would do to get us back on track. However, if I hadn't called him, I wouldn't have heard from him. I busied myself with work and pushed beneath the sand the changes taking place in him. I felt ready to move forward even if it was alone. Like a turtle I'd take it slow and steady.

January 2013

I was fifty-nine years old and still processing being single but married at the same time. I needed to focus on something other than myself and my failed marriage, so I decided to do a yearlong advanced master's program in clinical social work that would begin in the spring.

I spent the beginning of 2013 packing up the house, selling things, securing a realtor, and filling out mounds of paperwork for a short sale. There was no coming out ahead after the housing crisis; we were in line to lose a lot of cash. When I met with the attorney who would oversee it, he asked, "Where's your husband?" I wasn't quite sure what to say, so I told the truth. "Gary would not be very helpful at these proceedings." He took my hand in his. "Forgive yourself, Rose. There is no way you could have predicted this housing crisis. Just let it go." As he spoke, I thought to myself, that's exactly what I wanted to hear from Gary. I gave notice at work, and, having made the decision to attend Eastern Carolina University in Greenville, North Carolina, I secured an apartment close to campus.

Gary and I barely spoke, but when we did it was about renovations being done on our mountain home. We did not talk about divorce. I needed time to uncomplicate our lives, and deep down I believed he still loved me with all his heart. With little hope I held on to the belief that he would change.

April 2013

Just before the master's program started, my niece was getting married in Massachusetts. A day before I left for western North Carolina to pick up Gary, I called him and asked if he would pick up a few items for my arrival: skim milk, OJ, half and half, bread, butter, cheese, and pastry. I also asked him to launder a set of sheets and to clean the one room he had set up in the house. I knew there would be dust and dirt from the renovations he and my brother were doing.

As I was on the last stretch of the ten-hour drive, there was a huge accident causing bumper-to-bumper traffic. I no sooner navigated away from it than I was caught in a torrential downpour. By the time I arrived at our mountain home I was worn, weary, and hungry. It was 7:00 p.m.

As I drove up, I noticed my brother still working on the front deck. I was too tired to even say hello, and I was a little miffed that he was still working. He always started jobs late, so while it didn't surprise me that he was there, all I wanted was peace and relaxation. I did not want to engage in social conversation.

As I entered the house, my dog greeted me and then promptly threw up at my feet.

"Gary, what's wrong with Sneezy?"

"I don't know, what's wrong with him?" he asked.

"He just threw up!"

Gary promptly got down to the floor and proceeded to kiss and hug the dog. "What's wrong? What's the matter? Daddy loves you." I got no greeting.

I dropped my bags and headed to the refrigerator. I could at least have a glass of milk and a piece of toast. I stood aghast in front of the refrigerator, looking at Gary's half-empty whole milk container and leftover food wrapped in foil. He had not bought anything I asked for.

As he walked into the kitchen, I began my rant.

"Why didn't you buy what I wanted?"

With a face not registering what the big deal was, he replied, "You can have some of my milk. I could run down and get you something if you want."

Now this was more of the husband I knew, willing to make up for his mistake. But it didn't appease me. I knew that meant an hour of waiting until he returned home. I just resigned myself to being hungry. I would make up the bed and go to sleep.

As I grabbed the sheets Gary said he cleaned I noticed that they were twin sheets instead of the full sheets that would fit the bed. I also noticed that he had not cleaned the room, as there were layers of dust everywhere. It was this type of behavior that was partially responsible for our separation. Where once Gary was attentive to my needs, would welcome me home from a trip, take my bags and carry them into a room, and make sure there was food in the house, he appeared to not know what to do anymore. He was not bitter over the separation; in fact, I was not certain he even remembered I had asked for one. I had no intention or interest in chasing after this man while he sat back and made no effort.

I quickly dusted the room, threw dirty sheets in the washer, and grabbed my purse. My tears were my sole companion down that mountain, into town, to get takeout food. My hurting heart, exhaustion from the last year, and the need to stay focused on reentering college were front and center. There was no space in my mind to explore or care about Gary's change in behavior and his apathy toward us. I was just disgusted with it all.

Summer 2013

Gary would occasionally drive down to Greenville, North Carolina, to see me. Each time he came I was more alarmed, as his behaviors didn't match the man I married. Before one visit he sent me flowers. This was very unusual, as Gary was not a gift giver. I assumed he was trying to make up for lost time. I was startled by the bouquet he sent because it was very large, and I knew it must have cost a fortune.

When I heard a knock at the door and opened it, I found him standing outside looking anxious.

"Hi," I said.

He brushed past me. "Where are the flowers I sent?"

"Huh? They're in my bedroom," I said. "Why?"

He walked into the bedroom, looked at the flowers and became very angry.

"These flowers are horrible! These aren't what I ordered. I can't believe they screwed up."

I stood there totally puzzled. It was so uncharacteristic of Gary to be angry about anything. Least of all flowers. Plus, the arrangement was beautiful.

"Babe, what is wrong? They are beautiful."

He just shook his head and retreated to the couch.

I always used to tell everyone, "I swear I should put a mirror under Gary's nose to see if he's breathing." He was always so calm and showed no fire, so this behavior left me confused.

When I was first introduced to Gary, I had no interest in forming a relationship with him or anyone else. He was divorced, had a fourteen-year-old son, and, because he had assumed all marital debt, he had a lot of catching up to do. One day he shared the amount of debt he was carrying. I offered to create a budget for him. I told him, "I guarantee you if you'll follow it, you'll get out of debt." Having no money management skills, he readily agreed. His Master of Business Administration degree, which had honed his algebra and calculus skills, had done little to help him balance a checkbook.

On our dates we'd go Dutch. He'd look over at me. "Seriously. I'll pay."

"Babe, I've allocated no money in your budget for me. Just get out of debt. I refuse to redo your budget!"

"Okay," he'd say with sincerity. "I'll make it up to you."

I had recently returned from Italy, where I had been engaged to a man I referred to as my Italian Stallion. Aldo was handsome, outgoing, and very romantic. His main purpose in life was to have fun. Career, stability, trustworthiness, and saving money were further down on his list. Gary was the direct opposite.

What I learned to admire about Gary was his family commitment, honesty, kindness, listening ear, sense of humor, and deep commitment to humanity. His kindness extended to any living creature. Very often I'd catch him picking an insect off the floor in our house and carrying it outside.

"Really?" I'd question.

"It's just a little guy. He's not doing any harm."

Gary wasn't a gift giver. Unlike Aldo, who lived to surprise me with jewelry, flowers, and trips, this character trait was not in Gary's DNA. My first birthday gift was three t-shirts in a Walmart bag. They weren't even wrapped. I'm sure he got a discount as he worked there at night stocking shelves. He took a part-time job to be able to treat his son to outings on weekends after his divorce. There was no room in his budget for that.

Our relationship was quite different from temporary relationships, which reach a peak quickly and then subside. We were soul mates who shared everything with no jealousy over past relationships. I never heard him turn down a request for help from anyone, including me. The man literally never said *no*.

"Babe, I swear. When you die, I'm going to put 'Gary was sooooooo nice' on your tombstone."

He'd laugh. "Yeah, right."

"No," I'd say. "I'm gonna do it cuz that's all anyone ever says about you."

Gary was also very handy around the house. He was my handy dandy man. I'd often sing a jingle to him. "Gary, Gary, he's my man. If he can't do it, no one can."

He'd just laugh. "Okay, what do you need done now?"

The foundation of our relationship was friendship. And after six years of being each other's best friend, and after two marriage proposals declined by yours truly, I finally said "I do." I was afraid of losing my identity in marriage, or losing the freedom to explore different things, so I wrote words to reflect our views of what marriage signified. Gary was not a writer, but he readily agreed with what I wrote. Gary was not the type of man to hold me back from any dreams my heart held. He was always very supportive.

He was finally out of debt when we married, and I made it clear: I own the checkbook. I told him, "You can have anything you want, but I insist on managing our funds." He readily agreed. He trusted me explicitly. I feared if I did not manage our finances, Gary would put us in debt. Freedom from debt always meant *freedom* to do anything to me.

I gave my heart, and he gave his.

December 2013

In December Gary's brother passed away. Although Gary and John never shared a close relationship, he wanted to go to the funeral. "He's still my brother. My parents would want me to go." I was a little apprehensive because of the changes I was seeing. But I pushed back my fears. I told him, "Fine, make the reservations."

"How do I do that?" he asked. Gary was a worldwide traveler. Why didn't he know how to reserve a ticket? I convinced myself that he was just stressed over his brother's death, so I agreed to reserve the tickets. I had enough on my plate to contend with. I was six months short of earning my advanced master's degree. *He's fine*, I reassured myself.

Several hours into the trip I received a frantic call from Gary saying he missed his connection. He explained it wasn't his fault, as his initial flight took off late. The airline had another connection, but it was to a different airport than the one at which my brother-in-law was supposed to pick him up. Gary was lost as to what he should do.

Gary and I both traveled extensively with our careers and on vacations. He knew the ins and outs of airports, grabbing cabs, and making his way to his destination. Now he clearly did not know what to do. Was it stress? My gut was telling me different, and my earlier fears—which I did not want to welcome—resurfaced.

I phoned my brother-in-law about the flight change.

"Gary's plane got diverted. Can you pick him up in Massachusetts?"

"It's late. Have him grab a cab," he quickly responded.

I felt agitated. "You know there's something not quite right with Gary. You saw the changes in him. I'm not sure what is going on, but I know Gary will not be able to secure a cab."

"Well, I'm not driving over an hour away," he said sternly. "It's late, and I'm tired. You'll need to figure something out."

I hung up the phone feeling outraged by the lack of concern for a man he considered his best friend. I immediately thought of all the times Gary and I had helped his family. Gary was due to stay there for the week. Where would he stay now? I gathered my wits and called Gary's son. Ralph agreed to pick him up and drove his father to his home, where Gary stayed for the week.

May 2014

I completed my master's degree in social work and reviewed every choice I had to move on with my life. Gary was still at the mountain home, and the lease on my apartment in Greenville, North Carolina, was nearly up. I heard an inner voice gently persuading me to join Gary in western North Carolina. I forced it from my mind. I tried to reason with it. *But we are separated. I want to move on with my life.* I'd explain why it was not a good idea. But the voice persisted. *Go back.* The voice had a sense of urgency and convinced me of what I feared. That Gary left on his own was struggling to navigate his life. I told myself, *perhaps it's his seizure medication. I'll go to his providers and insist on answers.* Reluctantly I decided to return, rest, make sure that Gary was okay, and then put the house up for sale. I could not in good conscience leave him without a self-sufficiency toolbox.

My return home was not a surprise to Gary. His mind had simply dismissed my request for a separation. He walked into our bedroom the following morning, lay on my bed, and said, "I'm so happy to see you." My heart was happy at his sudden shift of attitude, but I was not convinced that the husband I married was now lying on my bed.

The first thing I noticed as I walked through the house was the stretch of beam that outlined my kitchen counter. I couldn't quite make out what was on it, so I moved closer. Side by side were toy cars. I picked one up, and it looked quite old. With my mouth half open, I looked at Gary.

"What's this?"

"That's one of the cars I had as a kid. I thought I'd display it."

I walked into the kitchen. I suddenly became curious as to what food he had brought into the house. I opened the tall cupboards that were used to store dry goods. I stared in disbelief at all his tools.

"What are your tools doing in our kitchen?"

"They are easier to get at," he replied. I stood there confused. The garage where his toolbox sat gave him easier access than the kitchen.

I peeked into an upstairs bedroom. Sitting in the middle of it was a futon chair he had brought with him. A makeshift crate serving as an end table sat beside it. I wasn't sure how to comprehend this. *Was this an attempt at decorating?*

I remembered two years earlier when he moved back here. He had spent days calling U-Haul for rental rates. He came and announced to me it would cost $3,000.

"Huh? What are you talking about? You are only taking a futon that will double as a bed, two nightstands, two lamps, DVD player, movies, the TV, and the stand it sits on. The boxes containing dishes, pots and pans, glasses, silverware, towels, linens, and toiletries won't take up a lot of room. Most of your tools are still at the mountain home. You can take whatever else you want, but all you need is a trailer to hook up to your hitch on your SUV."

I remembered him looking totally perplexed. It was as if suddenly the realization of his grossly misjudged calculation was registering. I found myself calling U-Haul, ordering a trailer, packing up his belongings, and waving goodbye to him from our driveway.

My friends did not understand my decision to return. They said, "You have no obligation to him." While that was true, I had noticed red flags in his behavior for over two years, and, although we hadn't been husband and wife for a while, I needed to make sure he was okay. If he wasn't alright, I wanted to help him figure out what to do. I could not desert a vulnerable human being who was incapable of finding his way out of an airport. Especially a man I considered my best friend.

He was a good man and a wonderful father to his sons. We shared many happy times, and vacations with nieces and nephews. He was a devoted son to his parents and watched over them until they both passed. He was there for my aunt when she needed help with home repairs. He never expressed displeasure with anyone. He loved to say, "Life is about people, babe." Although he might not have appreciated how someone behaved, he didn't let their behavior affect him. He'd never allow anyone to steal his peace. Because of the man he was, it was impossible for me to leave until I figured out why he was behaving so strangely.

Fall 2014

I began noticing more differences in behavior now that I was back living with Gary. I would find him playing solitaire for hours on his computer. His only other activity was walking the dog. Any suggestions I made for how he might spend his time were dismissed. If I joined him for a walk or tried to engage him in conversation, he would interrupt mid-sentence and talk about the dog. "Look at Sneezy, isn't he funny? Look at him running up those banks." His life appeared twofold. He had solitaire and his dog. It wasn't long before I stopped attempting to engage. I took this behavior to mean that he didn't want to make any attempt to improve our marriage. He was picking up right where he had left off.

We received tragic news that my great niece was seriously ill. We immediately flew out to Oregon in October and then again in November. I noticed Gary appeared totally lost in different environments. In the airport he took an inordinately long time emptying his pockets and gathering his things at security. Where once he navigated trips with ease, he constantly needed guidance on what to do. *Babe, show them your ticket. Don't forget your bag. Hurry up, we'll miss our connection. What do you want to eat?* My answer to my impatience was to direct and do as much as I could for him. It was easier than having to explain things.

One day he decided to take my niece's dogs for a walk. Soon after we received a call from her neighbor.

"There's a guy here that has your number on his phone. He says he's visiting but doesn't know where you live." Where alarm bells should have gone off, I dismissed them. *It's a new neighborhood*, I told myself. *He must have been distracted.*

My niece told me she had purchased some shelves that needed to be installed. I immediately volunteered Gary for the job. His handy dandy skills would put them up without any problem. Naturally, when I asked him, he said, "Sure." But it was impossible not to notice how he struggled using the tools. When finished, we noticed the shelves were installed incorrectly. I was unsure of what I was seeing. Gary had built sheds and sunrooms, renovated bathrooms, and installed stone foundations and tiles, and yet he had difficulty installing ready-made shelves.

At this point in the journey, I vacillated between wanting to help him and being consumed with self-pity over my own unhappiness. I just wanted him to behave the way I remembered. I felt certain others were seeing the changes in Gary, but no one offered any explanation. I didn't want to appear to be critical of him without having hard facts. I convinced myself as soon as we returned home, I would meet his healthcare providers and get answers. I was not anticipating any diagnosis other than age.

Summer 2015

Despite my promises to myself, I still had not met Gary's providers. I was tired of dealing with stuff and took some time to regroup from my studies and spend time with friends. However, in June, my hand was forced. My sister and her husband came to North Carolina to visit. We all decided to take a road trip to Nashville, Tennessee. After getting settled in a hotel, we visited local sights and attended the Grand Ole Opry. Gary seemed okay on the trip, a bit preoccupied, but otherwise content and happy.

We returned home late, and Gary and I retreated to our separate bedrooms. At nearly 10 a.m. the next morning, I noticed that Gary had not come downstairs. Gary had always been an early riser, so I was a little puzzled. Thirty minutes later he walked into the living room.

"You're up late," I said.

He stared at me.

"Are you okay?" I questioned.

"Yeah, I'm okay."

"Are you sure?" I implored.

"Yeah, I'm okay."

It felt silly at the time, and I'm not even sure what prompted me to ask, "Do you know who I am?"

"Yeah, I'm okay."

My anxiety started to rise. "Babe, you know who I am, right?"

"Yeah, I'm okay."

Panic gripped me. I directed him to a chair. I sat down on the floor in front of him. "Babe, no fooling around. You know who I am, right?"

"No. I don't."

I quickly ran into my bedroom, grabbed my car keys, and helped him to the car. As I drove to the ER in a torrential downpour, I asked him questions hoping to get a good response. His only response was "I'm okay."

At the ER, I informed the attending physician that I thought my husband was pre- or post-seizure. Gary had developed seizures in his teens when he crashed his motorcycle through a barbed wire fence. However, Primidone, an antiseizure medication, had kept them under control. I witnessed him having a seizure once, and I remembered that before he seized, he was repetitive in his speech.

The doctors began seizure medicine intravenously. Gary started to respond appropriately after an hour. The doctors felt he either had a breakthrough seizure or a grand mal seizure prior to coming downstairs. They decided to change his seizure medication of fifty years, from Primidone to Keppra. I was told Primidone was old and outdated and that there were better seizure medications on the market.

I learned that Gary had not seen a neurologist in years because his primary care provider prescribed his seizure medications. I researched and found a neurologist who would take Gary as a new patient. I reported to him all the behaviors I had seen over the last few years. After giving Gary a physical exam and a mini mental status exam (MMSE), the neurologist did not feel any other test was warranted to address Gary's recent behaviors. He said, "It's age and mood related." I was immediately relieved. *So, I had been correct, it was his age.*

I found a part-time position as a tutor and behavior interventionist at an elementary school and tried to resume my life. I was not moving anywhere until a reasonable amount of time passed and I was convinced that Gary could live independently. However, as the months wore on, I was growing more and more frustrated with his level of confusion, and now I was realizing he was losing his short-term memory. If I talked to him about visiting my dad the day before, he'd have no memory of going there. When we were at a festival, he could not find his way back to the parking lot. Gary had always had excellent recall. I promised him that I would find a doctor who would run some tests and figure out if something other than old age was causing these changes. If so, perhaps there were medications that could help.

Flashback

When I felt neglected during our marriage, I'd rant at Gary, "You never buy me anything! You know, a real gift. Wrapped with a bow. You know, a surprise. To show appreciation for everything I do."

To which he would reply, "You know how much I appreciate you! You own the checkbook. Buy yourself anything you want. You know I'd never stop you."

"But it's not the same!" I'd whine.

And so twice he purchased gifts to try and appease me. The first time he got me a skimpy negligee from Victoria Secret. I was well into my forties, and we had a nine-year-old son. Gary had the store wrap it beautifully in a box adorned with a big bow.

He stood there waiting. I prayed he didn't see the shock on my face. "Babe, this was very sweet of you to do. It's beautiful. Truly, honestly, I appreciate the thought, but I won't wear this. I mean, if you want me to wear it just in the bedroom, I will. I'll even try it on for you. But I can't walk around the house in this. Plus, I'll freeze my butt off."

"It's okay," he said. You can take it back."

I walked over and hugged him. "It was really a lovely thought. Thank you." Remembering this day, I should have just kept it. But in those days, with money limited, I was more conservative and used the refund to buy a nightgown I could wear more often. I know, boring!

The next gift was years later. It was a crucifix necklace with diamond chips. I wore a crucifix around my neck every day. It was gold with a single diamond. It was plain and simple. I never liked switching jewelry and leaving dressy pieces in a jewelry or safety deposit box. It made no sense to me. If it was pretty, I wanted to wear it every day.

Immediately Gary sensed something was wrong. "You don't like it?"

"Babe, I love it. I really do. But honestly, I won't wear it. Do you mind if I exchange it for something I'll wear more often?"

"No. Of course not. I want you to be happy."

The next day I went to the jewelry store and picked out simple silver and gold hoops. They were much more expensive than I'd ever purchase, but I matched what he paid for the cross. When I returned home, I showed them to him. I hugged him and said, "Thank you for my beautiful earrings and trying to purchase the perfect gift. I'll wear these earrings always."

I kept my promise. They grace my ears every single day. I also let the poor guy off the hook and never ranted again about him not buying me a gift. He was very grateful. He readily admitted, "I absolutely hate shopping. I love you, but I hate shopping." I thanked the Lord for such an understanding man.

First half of 2016

I kept encouraging Gary to go places while I was working, but he stayed close to home. If he went with me anywhere, he followed me around. This was so uncharacteristic of Gary, who always ventured off on his own. I phoned his neurologist and contacted his primary a few times explaining my concerns, but both felt his symptoms did not warrant a visit. They told me I needed to accept that Gary was getting older. Totally frustrated, Gary decided to try some supplements for memory improvement from a local Walgreens.

One afternoon I asked Gary to go to the grocery store. I had a sore throat and wanted a jar of honey and a bag of cough drops. He returned with honey cough drops. I also noticed that he was unable to do things that used to be second nature to him. I'd return home to find him sitting in the living room fiddling with the buttons on the remote control. The TV would be blank or snowy.

"Babe, why didn't you call the cable company to help you fix the problem?"

"I don't know," he'd reply. The fact was he could no longer find the contact list on his cell phone. He was now on his third phone, including the Jitterbug phone, which was kindergarten friendly. Despite my attempts to teach him how to use it, he could not remember the instructions.

He still drove, performed small chores around the house, and heated up food in the microwave. However, quite often I'd come home to find the kitchen filled with smoke. In the microwave I'd find a blackened piece of food. He had also developed a blank, out-of-focus look. I'd look at him shaking my head and say, "There's that blank look again." I wrote in on a list that I planned to take to his new neurologist.

One day I asked him to vacuum my car. Although the garage had an overhead light, he opted to use a car clamp light. He hooked it up to the inside handle above the door. It fell while he was vacuuming, resulting in a huge burnt hole in my leather seats.

I don't know why I kept asking him to do things despite his obvious limitations. It was not because I consciously thought he would fail. Perhaps it was so he would disprove what my gut could not label but was causing me anxiety. If the doctors felt he was okay, maybe I was just making more out of his older age than it was. Most times I asked him to do something, I just expected he could. They were such simple tasks. *He cannot possibly screw this up*, I thought.

My burnt seat infuriated me. I did what I do best when I am overtaxed: I screamed at him. I told him, "Just go, just go anywhere. I cannot take this anymore!"

I cried as he pulled out of the driveway. Tears of frustration. Tears of hurt. Tears of exhaustion of having to do everything in and around the house, working, and shouldering all the responsibilities that were once shared. When the tears stopped and I was calmer, guilt set in.

Why did I scream at him? What the hell is wrong with me? He's a good man. He just wasn't thinking. He can't help how he is. Part of me did not want to leave him alone to fend for himself, but another part wanted to board the next plane out. Seeing him every day made me miss the Gary I knew and loved. I missed talking to my best friend, laughing with him, or sharing a movie or dinner. We shared nothing that we once did. I had no idea what to do, so I alternated between wanting to help him navigate life or leaving. It was downright exhausting.

June 2016

In June Gary had his regular six-month checkup with his neurologist. Again, I went with a detailed list of everything I observed. The neurologist looked over the list and claimed his symptoms were again age related, mood, and epilepsy. I persisted. "No! Something else is wrong! I'm tired of this. I keep telling you he is not the same man, and you keep dismissing me." With a calm demeanor, the neurologist then suggested that perhaps his seizure medication was not at the correct dose.

He ordered an ambulatory electroencephalogram (EEG). It functioned like a normal EEG, but it was portable and would measure Gary's brain activity for a forty-eight-hour period. The results showed seizure activity during sleep, so the doctor upped Gary's seizure medication and put him on Aricept in hopes it would improve his memory and help with his processing. The short burst of hope I had that the recommended medication changes would work did not last.

A month later, Gary and my dad decided to fly to Rhode Island. While visiting my sister, Gary had an episode. Everyone was outside enjoying conversation. When they looked over at Gary, he was almost catatonic.

"Gary, Gary are you okay?"

He sat stoically, not responding.

They kept prompting him until he came around.

"Where am I? Where's Rose? he questioned.

"Gary, Rose did not come with you. Are you alright?" my sister asked. Alarm bells went off in her head, but she had no idea what to do.

She reported to me that he remained confused for quite some time. He kept asking her where I was because he did not believe I hadn't traveled there with him.

During that same visit, he drove to Vermont to visit his son. His son reported that Gary offered to help erect a tent for his granddaughter's high school graduation, but he was unable to execute the simplest steps. His son dismissed it, saying, "I'm sure Dad was just tired from the trip, but he was also more engaged with my dogs than with us." That surprised me, as Gary was always very sociable and looked forward to seeing his son's side of the family. I added both instances to a new list for the neurologist. Reflecting later, I'm sure dogs felt safer for Gary to be around. They provided love and did not expect anything in return. They also would not notice anything amiss in his behavior or make him feel embarrassed. He did not have to perform for the dogs. A dog's love is seen in their actions. I'm sure Gary was comforted by that. Later in this journey I wished people were more like dogs.

July 2016
We lose Sneezy

Sneezy was a rottweiler mix that my brother rescued. When my brother could no longer care for Sneezy, he passed him to my mom. When my mom passed, Dad gave Sneezy to Gary and me. Dad was never very fond of dogs.

Shortly after we got Sneezy, I took him to a veterinarian. I was told that a lot of his teeth were bad and were hanging by their nerve endings. They extracted nine teeth and found pieces of chain link fence embedded in his gums. The veterinarian believed as a puppy he chewed his way out of a chain he was tethered to.

I believe that is why Sneezy loved us so deeply. His beginning was so full of loneliness and abandonment that he would rather lose his teeth to a chain link fence than succumb to a life without love. Providing love was Sneezy's life's purpose.

When my dad brought him into our Wilmington home, Sneezy immediately found my other rescue, Rosie. Sneezy jumped into her bed. I expected Rosie to nudge him out or retreat elsewhere, but she welcomed him. Rosie was so independent and incredibly stubborn. But for reasons not apparent to me, both Rosie and Sneezy fell instantly in love.

When Rosie passed away two years later, Sneezy attached himself to us even more. He instinctively knew if he should be at our side or on his pillow. His back end would nearly detach itself from his body when we came home. It wagged back and forth so quickly and with such force you'd almost scramble to get out of its way.

Within an hour after Gary arrived home from his trip, I noticed droplets of blood on the floor and beads of blood around Sneezy's nose. I was not alarmed, as nine months before the same thing had happened. The x-rays the vet took found a tooth embedded in his sinus canal and extracted it. When I noticed the droplets, I immediately suspected another dental issue.

We decided to wait until morning, hoping the bleeding would subside. When it did not, I asked Gary to take him to the veterinarian and to call me when he knew something. I would be close by getting a haircut.

As soon as I arrived at my stylist, I received a call from the veterinarian.

"Sneezy has a serious issue. Your husband is terribly upset. Can you come over?"

Panic gripped my heart. I stammered, "Yes, of course. I'll be there in 10 minutes."

On the drive over I kept reassuring myself. After all, I just spent an entire week with Sneezy. He was perfectly okay.

When I entered the office, I noticed Gary sitting in a chair, pale and visibly shaken. I went over to provide comfort to him and then approached the front desk. The veterinarian soon joined us.

"Mrs. Jordan, I've never seen this in all my years of practice. Sneezy has zero platelets."

"Huh?" I scrambled around in my head for a definition of platelet.

"I don't understand," I stammered.

"I have seen dogs come in here with as low as 10,000 platelets. Sneezy has none. He is bleeding to death."

I could feel the tears welling in my eyes. "I don't understand. Sneezy isn't sick."

The veterinarian said, "I conferred with the doctor who saw him nine months ago. It's not a dental issue. We suspect a malignant nose tumor. You can put him in your car and drive him into Asheville. If he survives the trip, they will treat him with high dose steroids to stop the bleeding. I do not recommend it. We don't feel he will survive. Even if he does, and they can stop the bleeding, the tumor will need to be treated. He just doesn't have a good survival rate."

I could hear Gary whimpering. I fought to contain my emotions. *We must do what's best for Sneezy. How could this be happening? Oh my God, no.* I turned Gary.

"Babe, listen to me. Listen to me. We love Sneezy. We love him to death. But the best thing is to put him to sleep. We do not want him to suffer."

Gary emphatically shook his head no.

"We can do this, babe. Let's do what's best for Sneezy."

I went into the restroom and washed my face of tears. I began steeling myself to go in and see my dog.

The veterinarian approached me. "It's bad in there," she warned. "There's a lot of blood."

I directed Gary to come with me. As I entered, I found Sneezy lying in a pool of blood. I immediately got down on the ground beside him and laid my face next to his. Cradling his body, I looked into his eyes. They appeared to be pleading with me.

"It's okay, Sneezy. Mommy is here. It is going to be alright; I promise. I love you, Sneezy, so much. We are going to take care of you. Don't be afraid. Daddy's in here too."

I willed myself to appear strong for Sneezy. I stayed glued to the floor, nose to nose with a dog that I loved with all my heart and soul. And I stayed there until he took his last breath. Gary was holding the back end of him. This was my third dog I let go rather than allow him to suffer. I didn't know at the time that one day I would do the same for Gary.

When I got home, I wished that I could tear my heart out and put it on my desk to ease my tears. I walked zombie-like throughout the house, not knowing where to go or what to do. I finally grabbed a blanket, laid it by Sneezy's bed, and wrapped my arms around an empty hole.

The next morning, I woke up to a sense of dread. My Sneezy was gone. Gary's dog was gone. It was his lifeline when I was not home. I quickly remembered that we had forgotten his collar, and I dialed the clinic. After explaining my dilemma, they told me they would search the office and phone me back.

A few hours later I got an apologetic call from the veterinarian. She told me it had never happened before, but they searched every inch of the building and could not find his collar. She assumed it was cremated with him.

There were more tears and then a boost of determination. I searched our vehicles inside and out and combed every square inch of our home. More tears and then quiet resignation. Sneezy's collar and his scent were gone.

A few weeks later I awoke praying as I lay in bed. I quietly spoke to Sneezy.

"Sneezy," I began, "It's mom. You know how much I loved you, how much I still do, but Mommy really needs to get another dog for Daddy. He's so very sad. And you know with his memory failing and being here alone most days, he really needs a doggie. So Sneezy, if you want Mommy and Daddy to have another doggie, please find him for us."

I then got up and announced to Gary that we were going down to the shelter. We would just peek at the dogs that were available. Once there, I told the man in charge to let four dogs I had selected out of their cage and into the yard. I wanted to see if any came to me.

Immediately a black lab mix ran up to me with his back end going from side to side just like Sneezy. Gary and I played with him, and he seemed like a nice dog. I told the man we would think about it and let him know.

I spent the rest of the day thinking about him. Gary did as well. The next morning, as I lay in bed, I again talked to Sneezy.

"Sneezy," I began, "It's Mom again. I found another doggie, Sneezy. I think he is the one. Can you please send me a sign if this is the dog you have chosen for us?"

After having some coffee and getting dressed, I convinced myself that Gary and I should go to the shelter and take another look. I asked my husband to go out to the SUV and bring in Sneezy's leash. I had never removed it from the car.

I said, "If we decide to bring the dog home we'll have to stop at Walmart and get a collar, as I don't have Sneezy's anymore."

About five minutes later, Gary walked in with the leash in one hand and Sneezy's collar in the other. What? I stood there dumbfounded.

In disbelief I asked, "Where did you get that collar?"

Gary responded, "It was on the back seat of the SUV."

"That's impossible," I said. "I take the SUV nearly every day to the lake and I lay my raft on the back seat. I would have seen it! Don't you remember? We searched both cars after Sneezy died looking for his collar."

He looked puzzled as he said, "I found the collar lying next to the leash on the back seat." I didn't know what to think. *Maybe I was going crazy too.*

2017

Work was becoming more and more of an escape. Gary was withdrawing and began losing weight. The scale confirmed a ten-pound drop. I phoned the neurologist, who attributed it to the Aricept he prescribed. Instead, he placed Gary on memantine, which the doctor felt would help with Gary's articulation. Gary was now having difficulty articulating his thoughts. He was constantly searching for the right word to use.

I immediately saw an improvement in Gary's language after he started the medication. Still, the doctor offered no clue as to why Gary was experiencing these symptoms. *Is this old age too? Would I one day not be able to form a sentence?* It made absolutely no sense to me, but I was not a neurologist.

I suggested to the doctor that Gary be placed back on his old seizure medication. "Maybe it's the Keppra. He never had these difficulties on Primidone." But the neurologist vetoed it. He said, "Primidone is an old medication, they don't even use it anymore for seizures. His new seizure medication would not cause any of the symptoms he's having." He appeared to know more about what was not causing the changes than what was.

At 7:30 a.m., before I left for work, I would always make sure Gary was up. I'd leave him sitting on the couch watching TV and eating a bowl of cereal. I'd make sure he had taken his medications. I had realized months earlier that he was not taking his pills as directed, so I put myself in charge of managing his medication.

The only time Gary ventured out was with Chase. We lived on a mountain ridge, and Chase would always manage to get out of his choker collar. Chase wouldn't go very far and would always come home, but it caused Gary a great deal of anxiety. Some days I'd pull up to the house and hear Chase barking. If I looked down our driveway, I would see Chase sitting under a tree looking up at a squirrel, barking his foolish head off. And there would be Gary, leash in hand, trying to coax him back. I'd roll down my window and try to reassure Gary, "Just

What is wrong with my husband?

let him be, he'll tire and come home." But Gary would remain fixated on Chase. As I pulled into the garage, I wondered how long he'd been standing out there.

One day I gave him a list of calls to make. One was to the insurance company and another was for needed repairs to the house. I listed the phone numbers and wrote out steps one, two, and three of what I wanted him to ask. When I returned home, he told me he had not called. I sat next to him and encouraged him to call.

"Come on, babe. You can do this. Just follow the list of instructions."

He became frustrated halfway through because he could not articulate his thoughts or process the information quickly enough. I reached for the phone and completed the call. Another thing to put on the list for the neurologist. Surely if I kept providing clues, the doctor would have a better idea what was going on. My father was fifteen years older than Gary, and he wasn't having these issues.

Some other things I noticed. Gary and I preferred different things to eat. For lunch he preferred a tuna fish sandwich, a bowl of soup, or canned ravioli. I made sure that when I shopped, he was well stocked. I began noticing that his food remained untouched. OMG, he was not remembering to eat!

The one job Gary always had throughout our marriage was setting up the coffee pot at night. But often when I woke up, I found it had not been set up. When he did remember to prepare it, I'd find coffee all over the countertop and floor. He had either overfilled the machine with water or put the coffee in without the filter. I would begin my morning ranting while cleaning up the mess before hurrying to work. I knew if I left it to Gary the cleanup would not be done properly.

My behavior was not something I was proud of, and I'd spend days feeling guilty about it. *Stop it, Rose. Why are you yelling at him? Something is wrong.* It was quite awful. Behaving poorly. Feeling guilty. Being good for a few days. Behaving poorly again. I was emotionally tired from dealing with it and physically exhausted from the additional workload. I felt I was getting nowhere in moving on with my life or helping Gary. Anger, bitterness, frustration, and impatience started rising in me. My desire to help Gary was wearing thin. Other than taking him to appointments and tracking observations, I had no idea what else to do. The doctors who should have been listening to me were not.

Family members did not lend emotional support. Their solution was, "Quit your job." I told them, "It's the only JOY in my life," but they did not understand. "Well then," they'd say, "I don't know what to tell you."

Gary continued his neurologist and primary care appointments. Despite the growing list of behavior changes I was reporting, the examination continued to be the same. The neurologist would have him take his finger and reach for his nose (coordination good). He'd note his hand tremor but dismiss it. Then he'd have him walk across the room.

"It's not Parkinson's," he'd say. "I'd see it in his gait."

He'd then perform another MMSE (mini mental status exam) designed to evaluate everyday mental skills. It required Gary to answer a series of questions. Afterwards, the doctor wrote down the same diagnosis. Gary's condition was due to mood and age. I was ready to punch a hole in his wall.

I looked at him and said, "Gary doesn't remember our wedding day!"

"Now that's not right," he replied.

"Of course it's not," I said. "So, what's your answer? Or are you going to tell me it's age, mood, and/or his seizure medication yet again? This is ridiculous!" My patience was stretched to the max with medical professionals who simply did not listen. The doctor just stared at me with a totally blank look on his face. "I guess I can order another ambulatory EEG." I walked out totally frustrated. I wanted to tell him where to stick his EEG. I was losing my mind.

I was not able to compute this disconnect between a medical professional and a layperson. I was taught to document symptoms so the doctor had a starting point. Why was Gary's neurologist not taking advantage of the information I was providing? Was Gary's presentation so different from my reports that he did not believe me? A neurologist studies patients whose brains are damaged. Why did he not feel Gary's behaviors indicated some miswiring in his brain? If I could not depend on a medical professional to help find the answer to Gary's challenges, what was I to do?

Flashback

Memories of our engagement and wedding filled my mind. I looked down at my engagement ring—a gold rose with a diamond in the center. I remembered sharing the story with Gary about my previous engagement ring from Aldo, which was also a rose with a diamond. I sadly explained how devastated I was when it was stolen. Gary felt so bad. He made sure he found a jeweler to create another ring made with a rose and diamond before he proposed. The setting was not at all similar, but I fell in love with it immediately.

As I twisted the ring around my finger, memories surfaced of our wedding night. Out of debt, Gary had saved enough money for a down payment on a house. I chipped in the other half. We decided to have our wedding in our new home. November 8, 1986. I chose the month and day to honor my Nana, who had passed June 20 of that same year. It was her birthday.

I never desired a big wedding, and I knew my parents could not afford one. I bought a dress from a clearance rack and hired a caterer for hot hors d'oeuvres, a bartender, and an organist to play and sing our song, "You Needed Me" by Anne Murray. I had a cake made by a local cake lady. It was pink with a beautiful dove perched on top. A minister read the words we chose on what a marriage should be. The total cost of our wedding was $1,000.

Part of our vows read: A good marriage is a relationship of love. To be in love means to have a deep sense of identification with another person. It is to live in the life of that person, feeling his or her joys and troubles as if they were your own. And when two people are truly in love, each is concerned with helping the other become what he or she ought to be. The husband wants to nourish the best qualities of his wife; the wife wants to develop what is good in her husband.

The celebration had twenty-five invited friends and family, with Gary's son as best man and my sister as maid of honor. At 7 p.m., with the house illuminated by candlelight and vases of flowers everywhere, Gary and I became man and wife.

Gary was very concerned about what he needed to do during the ceremony. I calmed his fears and told him, "Nothing. You will just say the standard 'with this ring, I thee wed.'" But when it came time for that romantic moment, Gary became tongue tied. "With this *wing*, no I mean *wing*, **ring** I thee wed." I almost peed my pants, I laughed so hard.

June 2017

I scheduled another appointment with Gary's primary doctor. After reviewing everything with him, I begged him to tell me what more we could do to get answers for Gary's confusion, limited processing, and difficulty with language. The second ambulatory EEG had shown nothing new. Surely there was a test that could give us more clues on what was happening. It had been three years since I returned to our mountain home, and we did not have an answer that satisfied either one of us. Gary was becoming more and more upset with his diminished capacity to do things, and his self-esteem was also suffering.

His primary doctor looked me square in the eye and said, "Maybe it's *you* that has the problem."

I gathered my things, took Gary's arm, and stormed out of there. *You misogynistic fool*, I mumbled. *What was wrong with these doctors who did not listen and who could not suggest any tests to give us a clue as to what was going on? Did he believe I was imagining things? Making things up? Maybe I should introduce these doctors to an older man like my dad.* How many more professionals were going to insist that nothing was wrong with my husband? I had a clinical social worker degree and was trained in solution-focused therapy, and I had not a clue how to find a solution to this problem.

Life continued. I felt I had no choice but to stay and observe. I walked Gary over to weeds one afternoon and instructed him to pull them out the following day. He readily agreed, as he was constantly asking me to give him something to do so he'd feel useful. I was reluctant to give him a chore, fearing he'd screw up. But what could he possibly do wrong with weeds? When I returned home from work, I noticed he had pulled up all my beautiful perennials. I added another clue for the neurologist to my list. I went into my bedroom so Gary would not see my tears of frustration.

Another afternoon I returned home during a rainstorm. Gary was pacing through all the rooms.

"What's wrong?" I asked.

He yelled, "Something is trying to get into the house!" He was literally shaking, throwing up his hands, and appeared exhausted from trying to figure out what he was hearing.

I didn't understand. "What? I don't understand, babe. It's raining outside. We have no windows open."

He became even more visibly shaken. "Water, water is coming into the house! I don't know where it's coming in. I must find it!"

I did my best to calm him down, but it wasn't until the rain stopped that he stopped pacing through every room in the house, petrified.

On yet another occasion, I pulled into the driveway and noticed an extension cord extending from the garage door, across the driveway, and leading into the woods. When I got into the house, Gary was sitting on the couch.

"What's the extension cord doing in the driveway?"

"There's a tree root I want to chain saw off because it's sticking up from the ground. I'm afraid someone will trip over it."

I went down to the basement, found the chainsaw, and hid it.

Another time he was frustrated because he could not get the riding mower started. I told him to just leave it and said I'd ask my brother to come take a look at it. As I walked into the garage, I noticed he had started it inside. I smelled the smoke, and the whole back wall of the garage where the mower was parked was covered in oil. I had just painted it the day before. He had put oil in the gas tank and overfilled the oil compartment. His actions frightened me, and I feared for his safety. I had no idea what he might do while I was at work.

To cheer us both up I invited my six-year-old great-nephew over. Jason was so much fun, and he would have such patience with Gary. I had a tote box full of games, books, plastic soldiers, toy tanks and planes that would keep Jason busy for hours. I'd tell him, "Go play with Uncle." Within minutes Gary came into the kitchen pouting.

"What's wrong?" I'd ask.

"Jason is cheating. I can't play with a cheater."

I'd just stare at him. His behavior was reverting to that of a child.

To keep Gary busy when I was at work, I purchased a wooden model car kit. It was age appropriate for eight- to ten-year-olds. I thought because he loved cars and putting things together, it might provide some entertainment. Gary struggled with it for days. He could not get the wheels on properly. He then had the task of painting it and putting stickers on. I stared at the finished results; it looked like a second grader had put it together.

Thinking back, knowing what I know now, I feel rather stupid. But I was so ignorant of any diagnosis that would explain these behaviors. Obviously, the medical professionals he was seeing didn't know anything, either.

July 2017

Despite not having any answers, my need to move on with my life prompted me to begin looking for an apartment for him. The house was now market-ready, and I secured a realtor. But every time I found a place that might be suitable, I was stuck with the realization that I would need to clean, shop, cook, cover doctor appointments, and manage more finances if he moved. Gary was incapable of doing these things for himself. I found myself getting more and more depressed. I felt stuck in a situation I had no control over.

When Gary returned one afternoon after going into town, he told me about a building that was being constructed. Construction was always a passion of Gary's, so it did not surprise me when he said he hung around and talked to the construction crew. I was just happy he went out. I saw a brochure of an assisted living place lying on my desk.

"Huh, what is this?" I asked.

"It's that building that's being constructed. I like it. I want to live there."

I did not understand. "But it's assisted living! Do you know what assisted living is? You don't need assisted living!" I had a hard time comprehending a solution so drastic when we still did not know what was causing these changes. I still believed that Gary could be fixed if we found someone who knew what they were doing. I didn't realize at the time that Gary knew more about Gary than I did.

"I like it," he replied.

I was at a loss for words. I took the brochures and placed them in my inbox with no further discussion.

December 2017

By year end I knew that, despite what his neurologist was saying, I had to do something else to get a diagnosis. The day before Christmas I found a plastic bag in the garage. Curious, I looked in it. It was two plastic bushes of gravesite flowers.

I confronted him, "Is this my Christmas gift?"

He replied, "I wanted to get you flowers but they didn't have any in the store." On Christmas Eve, the time of year when there's an abundance of flower arrangements and poinsettias, Gary went to a store that sold plastic gravesite flowers and bought me a gift. I wish I could write that I controlled my anger that night. I did not. Beside my anger, all my previous feelings of being neglected resurfaced. I was shouldering so much responsibility, and he couldn't even pick me up a bouquet of flowers. What the hell was going on? What was wrong with him?

My emotions were all over the map. One minute I'd feel the emotional neglect that caused me to ask for a separation. The next minute I was angry that he screwed up. Then I'd cry because I felt sorry for him or felt guilty. Other times self-pity was my friend. Every day there was a new emotion I needed to regulate. Whether it was frustration and anger at the doctors, not being able to move on with my life, or feeling inadequate to get answers for Gary, I struggled day in and day out to find peace, all the while shouldering the full responsibility of a large home, finances, looking after my dad, and working.

After tearfully speaking with my niece, she suggested I take Gary to see a neuropsychologist. I had no idea how that would be helpful. Gary didn't need therapy. My niece encouraged me to make an appointment. I searched the internet and found one an hour and a half away. I was able to get an appointment in February 2018.

Dementia diagnosis

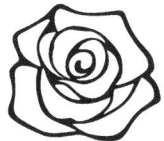

"There are moments
Which mark your life.
Moments when you
Realize nothing will ever
be the same and time is
divided into two parts,
before this, and after this.
Sometimes you can feel
Such a moment coming.
That's the test, or so I
tell myself. I tell myself
that at times like that,
strong people
keep moving forward anyway,
no matter what they're
going to find."

DENZEL WASHINGTON
as John Hobbes, 1998, "Fallen"

February 2018

The appointment with the neuropsychologist would take three hours. I couldn't imagine what he would do in that length of time, but I was praying for an answer to Gary's problem. His neurologist had no explanation, and I honestly could not imagine what a neuropsychologist would tell us.

We arrived at the office promptly. After the doctor came out and introduced himself to both of us, he asked Gary to remain in the lobby while he talked with me privately. Once in his office, he reviewed Gary's medications and medical history. He asked me what brought us there. I began explaining to him the changes I had seen in Gary's behavior in the last few years. He asked many questions, took notes, and asked me to bring Gary into his office. He told me to return in a couple hours while he performed some tests.

When I returned, Gary was still in his office. Within ten minutes I was ushered in. The neuropsychologist began reviewing all of Gary's test results. These included the Halstead-Reitan Neuropsychological Test Battery (Heaton, et al., 2004 norms), Reitan-Klove Sensory-Perceptual Examination, Boston Naming Test, and Trail Making Tests.

Gary's mental status was much lower than expected for his age and education. He faltered in naming the president and was not able to recite the months of the year backward. He set the hands of a clock face incorrectly, and although he recognized line drawings, he did not remember them after a brief delay.

His concentration, attention, and speed varied across different subsets, and he declined rapidly when he tried to multitask. His recall of a sixteen-item word list was significantly impaired, and he was moderately slower than men of his age and education in connecting numbered areas across a standard page. The rapid decay of his memory was very striking.

The neuropsychologist assured me he would study the results further but was ready to give a preliminary diagnosis.

Major neurocognitive disorder, suspected Alzheimer's disease.
This is an important part of our journey because early diagnosis is the key to seeking treatment. It took four years to get a diagnosis for Gary. Sadly, for whatever reason, caregivers spend years going from doctor to doctor without getting a diagnosis. Caregiver support groups attest to this every day of the week. I was diligent in attending neurologist and primary doctor appointments, and none of them ever suggested going to a neuropsychologist for further testing.

Inequities in access to the healthcare system and delays in diagnosis mean that even proven treatments are not necessarily helpful. The recently developed dementia drug Lecanemab must be given in early stages of dementia for it to be effective. It costs $26,500 without insurance coverage. With Medicare it will cost consumers about $5,000 a year ($416 a month).

When I heard the word Alzheimer, I felt shocked, confused, and scared all at once. The mixed feelings made me lightheaded, and I gripped the sides of the chair to steady myself. I felt anxiety and fear creeping into my gut. *Steady yourself, Rose—steady yourself. Don't look upset. Gary might pick up on it. Remain strong and in control. He's counting on you to understand this for him and ask the right questions.* My brain struggled to stabilize my emotions. I looked over at Gary's face to gauge what he was feeling in this exact moment. His face registered a flat affect, a lack of any emotion. *Okay, that's good*, I reassured myself. *He's not understanding this diagnosis.*

I said to the doctor, "Excuse me. I think I misheard you. What did you say?" He repeated the diagnosis, and I sat with questions forming in my mind.

"You said *suspected* Alzheimer's?" My mind relaxed. *Perhaps this was a mistake.*

The doctor continued. "Gary appears to only have one marker for Alzheimer's. I suspect he has vascular dementia. Primidone, the epilepsy medication Gary took for years, is probably the culprit. They don't even use it anymore because it has so many red flags for dementia. The solvents he worked around in the laboratory didn't help. Or it could be the head trauma he suffered in his twenties, which caused his seizures is rearing its ugly head. He's fortunate that he is just now feeling the effects from all this and that he's been able to accomplish so much in his life."

Huh? That didn't make me feel any better. I doubted anyone would call Gary fortunate.

I was ignorant about dementia or Alzheimer's. I thought they were one and the same. I did not know that Alzheimer's was just one of over one hundred forms of dementia. The most common are Alzheimer's, vascular, frontotemporal, and Lewy bodies. At the time I thought, *okay, he'll have a little memory loss. But I can manage some things for him.* I wasn't thinking of all the other behaviors I had been observing.

I asked Gary to wait in the lobby while I spoke to the doctor. I began, "As you know, I've been separated from Gary, and I'm looking for an apartment for him. So, does this mean that's not an option?"

"I'm not sure. Gary will need quite a bit of help, and he shouldn't be left alone for a long period."

I tried to digest what this would mean for my life. My gut was in a sudden knot. "No, wait. Gary and I are separated. We haven't been husband and wife for nearly seven years! You are not suggesting that we live together forever. Just how much will I need to do for him?"

"That's up to you," he began. "But Gary is not going to be able to function long on his own. Does he by any chance have long-term insurance?"

I took a minute to process his question and then remembered. "Yes, he does. But I don't know anything about it. I don't understand. Why are you asking me this?"

He replied. "That's your answer. They will pay for assisted living."

"My answer?" I stared at him blankly. "Assisted living?"

"It's the perfect time. I'm not sure what you are waiting for."

The realization of what he was saying hit me like a ton of bricks. My mind began racing. *Does this mean that Gary can't be self-sufficient just because of memory loss? What is going on? I need to get out of here and do research. I'm not sure what this man is talking about. I may be scared for no reason.*

I had one more question before I left. "What does this mean in terms of life span?"

"I predict Gary has five years," he replied. My face registered disbelief.

I took Gary to lunch, and I watched him more closely than I ever had before. I noticed that I asked him what he wanted, and then I ordered lunch for both of us. *How long had I been doing that? When was the last time we went out to eat that he ordered for us?*

Gary had always been so independent and self-sufficient. Suddenly I became aware that I had been filling in the blanks for him the last few years. When I wasn't yelling at him for screwing up, I was covering for him, believing he might not notice his lack of proficiency. I loved him. I would never want him to feel inadequate or embarrassed. Perhaps another reason I did it was denial or impatience with him.

I ordered Gary iced tea and handed him a cup. There was an iced tea machine nearby. As I was preparing my iced coffee, I looked over at Gary. He was standing with the cup in his hand, not knowing what to do. I walked over and without saying a word helped him put ice in the cup and then filled it with iced tea. *When was the last time he got his own drink?* I could not recollect. I walked to the table shaken. *How much had I been doing for him?* I knew why I was so worn and always on edge. I had been living the life of two.

I watched Gary eat. I didn't know how to talk to him about this. I felt sick to my stomach. I felt like crying and running out of the restaurant, but I don't run from challenges.

I began. "So, babe, we finally got a diagnosis of dementia."

I received no response.

"The doctor said that maybe assisted living would be good for you. What do you think?"

"Yeah, that would be okay. I liked the place I found."

Dementia diagnosis

I sat and stared at him. I waited for resistance. Any emotion to let me know he was upset by the diagnosis or moving to assisted living. I received nothing.

"Do you have any questions?"

"No," he replied.

"Do you know what this diagnosis means?"

He didn't respond.

He continued to eat his sandwich. He did not appear upset at all. The diagnosis did prove that Gary loved me. His lack of compassion, joy, sharing, apathy, emotional neglect, and physical distance from me had nothing to do with me. It was all attributable to this insidious disease. I realized that ranting and yelling at him in anger was easier than thinking he no longer loved me. The diagnosis soothed the emotional hurt I had felt for the last seven years, but, at the same time, guilt settled in. *How could I have not known that Gary was not responsible for his behavior? I should have known better and known his love would always be steadfast.* I knew from this point forward I would be kinder and gentler with him.

Some Facts About Dementia

Dementia is no longer an old person's disease. You can receive a diagnosis at any age. There is no significant incident rate between men and women and who will develop the disease at any given age. Dementia is not just memory loss. It affects personality, processing, and cognition until ultimately the brain fails completely and the patient dies. There is no cure.[1]

There are 5.8 million Americans that suffer from it; and it is projected by 2050 that 14 million will be coping with the disease in the United States. Fifty million people are living worldwide with some form of dementia, and rates may exceed 152 million by 2050. The worldwide cost of dementia is estimated to be 2 trillion by 2030.[2]

Alzheimer's is the sixth leading cause of death among all age groups and the fifth leading cause of death for people over 65.[3]

---

1. Alzheimer's Association, *2019 Alzheimer's Disease Facts and Figures*, https://alz.org/media/Documents/alzheimers-facts-and-figures-2019-r.pdf
2. *2019 Alzheimer's Disease Facts and Figures*; Hebert, "Alzheimer's Disease in the United States (2010–2050)"; Patterson, *World Alzheimer Report 2018*.
3. Melonie Heron, "Deaths: Leading Causes for 2016," *National Vital Statistics Reports* 67, no. 6 (2018): 1–77, online at https://www.cdc.gov/nchs/data/nvsr/nvsr67/nvsr67_06.pdf.

Ombudsman

After looking up data on the internet about dementia, my heart sank. This was not at all what I expected. As the disease progressed, Gary would not be able to read, write, process TV, dress himself, shave, or brush his teeth. He would be incontinent, need assistance with feeding, and eventually might not be able to swallow. He may become violent. *Gary? The meekest and mildest man I've ever known?* None of it seemed possible.

I got up from my desk. *This cannot be right.* I walked around the house. My mind and emotions were all over the place. *Surely this cannot be happening. No, this is all wrong. It MUST be something else. This can't happen to Gary. No, no, no. He doesn't deserve this!*

I remembered the neuropsychologist's words: "Gary has about five years left." We were in the seventh year since symptoms began. *Focus, Rose, focus.* Try as I might, the tears flowed. I felt myself gagging with the realization of it. I picked up a glass sitting on my desk and flung it across the room. I watched the glass shatter onto the tile floor. That was Gary's life, I thought. *Dementia will steal him piece by piece.*

I found Gary's long-term insurance policy. When he initially took it out and I learned that his premium was $350 a month, I was angry. That was higher than his Medicare, United Health, and my medical insurance combined. I wanted to cancel the policy when we were supporting two homes. I was now happy that I hadn't. I reached for the phone and left a message asking them to call me.

The next call I made was to a regional ombudsman. I knew from my social work education that they were the ones who took complaints from people residing in assisted living, memory care, and nursing homes. I was certain they could give me some directions on how to proceed. An ombudsman answered the call promptly and agreed to meet me the next day. I scheduled the appointment for after work and Googled the directions to his office.

Harry was around my age and welcomed me into his office. I told him about Gary and our meeting with the neuropsychologist. I handed him the report and gave him time to read it. I discussed with him the suggestion of Gary going into assisted living. I was convinced that he would tell me it was not necessary and that with a little help Gary would be fine in an apartment.

He began by sharing that he had cared for his parents. Both had dementia before they passed. As he told his story, I felt my heart sinking to the floor. He was confirming everything I had read.

I started to explain. "But Gary is not there yet! After our home sells, maybe I set him up in an apartment and help him manage things."

He looked at me sympathetically. "Perhaps, Rose, for six months, possibly a year. After that he will need more assistance."

"Are you suggesting that he live with me, and I take care of him?" *This was so much more than I had agreed to when I returned.*

"No, Rose, that is not what I am suggesting. You are already weary and tasked. I saw it the minute you entered this office. You need to listen and trust me. **You cannot do this alone.**"

"But . . ."

"Listen to what I am saying. It almost killed me, Rose. And I have spent a lifetime helping families care for loved ones with dementia. I am very knowledgeable about the disease. I counseled for years before I took on this job. **You cannot do this alone!** Most caregivers die before a person with dementia from the stress and the physical wear and tear. Caregivers get ill after the journey because they neglect their health for years. They are virtual prisoners in their home 24/7. They cannot leave the loved one they are caring for. Not even for a walk around the block. If you have long-term insurance, use it now. Get Gary settled so that he will feel safe and secure until the time comes when he'll know little else but the room he is staying in."

I felt dizzy and nauseous. I gripped the handles of the chair for support. I was unable to move. I took deep breaths. I began counting to ten. I felt my life being drained out of me. And then the floodgates of loss, despair, weariness, confusion, grief, and disbelief opened. I sat there unable to stop crying. I wanted to drown the room with my sorrow for Gary.

I heard Harry exit the room and looked up when he reentered with a box of tissues. He placed it in front of me as I continued to weep. He sat there motionless. He said nothing. After what seemed like a very long time, I got up to leave. He handed me a card for memory care. He explained it was a nonprofit organization about an hour away. Its staff would examine Gary, perform quarterly tests, and track his progress. They would also be there for me and our sons should we have any questions.

When I returned home, I took Harry's other advice and bought Gary a medical alert bracelet, which shared his name, address, and medical condition. I also bought a lifeline that he could wear around his neck. With an application installed on my phone, I could track him should he become lost. If he remembered, he could push the 911 button for instant help. I also gathered items he wore and put them in a plastic bag. As Harry explained, if he became lost, a rescue dog would be able to pick up his scent from his clothes. People with dementia wander, become lost, and are often found dead.

After diagnosis

"Empathy is really the opposite of spiritual meanness.
It's the capacity to understand that every war is both won and lost.
And that someone's else's pain is as meaningful as your own."

BARBARA KINGSOLVER

Animal Dreams

March 2018

I notified our sons, Ralph and Steve, and mailed them the report from the neuropsychologist. I also provided a copy of Gary's healthcare POA, which included them. I sent the contact information of a memory care specialist that would track Gary quarterly on this journey. Investing $700 a year for a specialist seemed worthwhile. I made sure both sons understood I would be available to answer any of their questions. In addition, I phoned a sibling whom I knew would inform the others of Gary's diagnosis.

I assumed that after notifying everyone of the diagnosis I'd have listening ears, occasional calls, and offers of physical help during a crisis. I felt certain they would call Gary and offer love and support, especially since he was now on borrowed time. They would want to visit, share memories, and offer hugs. Both sides of our family loved Gary. He never had a conflict with anyone.

The few people who called questioned the diagnosis and did not agree with Gary's decision to transition to assisted living. They thought that it was too soon, even though they had no basis for that opinion. One son questioned how it would be paid for. These were not the responses I had hoped for or expected.

One niece who was very close to Gary called and expressed her support and concern. She sent him a memory jar to record his memories. Gary wrote only four messages for the jar. In his scrawled handwriting he wrote:

I will look for the little snake in the garage on Thursday.
Nice call from Val 8:00 p.m. March 22, Thursday.
Chase misses his mom and will see her this weekend.
I will always remember my days with my wife Rose and dog Chase in Fontana Lake estates.

I mentioned to Gary that I hadn't heard from anyone. He stood up and began to cry. I was caught off guard, as crying was so uncharacteristic of Gary. His shoulders were hunched, and his tears flowed uncontrollably.

"OMG. What's wrong?" I asked.

"Is everybody going to throw me away?" He was now shaking as he cried.

In the years I had known this man, I had never seen him cry like this. During movies with animals or children, both of which he was sensitive to, I would look over to see tears rolling down his face. But rarely would he shed a tear in a real-life situation. I used to joke with him, "For someone with as big a heart as yours, you rarely show emotion."

I took his arm and guided him back to the couch. "Sit down. Look at me," I said.

He could barely meet my eyes, he was so distraught.

I began, "Listen to me, babe. I will never throw you away. Do you hear me? I will always be here. Do you understand?"

"Yes."

I continued. "I do not know why we've not heard from anyone. We will not worry about this right now. But I need you to know. I will always be at your side. Even when you no longer know I am there, I will be. I promise I will *never* abandon you."

I surprised myself with my own words. Hadn't I separated from this man and decided to return only until I found out what was wrong with him? Now I found myself committing my life to him. But I knew at that moment my decision to watch over Gary was based on love for another human being. We had lost the love that is shared between husband and wife. But he was a good and kind man and deserved to be cared for, watched over, and loved as any human should be. However, I had absolutely no idea what I had just committed to and the huge responsibility my words held.

I did not assume the caregiver role because I was an expert on dementia. I did not have extra time on my hands, and I had many other responsibilities. I did not feel I was stronger than other family members. It was not because I felt responsible for Gary. And lastly, I did not consider that my master's in social work would give me an edge in managing his care. I simply *cared for and loved* him.

When Gary brought home the brochures on assisted living in 2017, he knew what he would need. He did not want to burden me. At different times in our marriage, we would discuss what we would do if one of us became critically ill. Gary would always respond, "Do what you can but do not make yourself sick." He knew that his processing ability and memory were hindering his ability to remain independent. It was not in his nature to ask me to sit home and babysit or entertain him. So, while he was still able, he made this decision for himself. It's probably the most unselfish and loving decision anyone can make.

From my memory jar

Gary: "I saw you on your way to work today."

Me: "You did?"

Gary: "Yes. As I was passing your car, I noticed your window down. Your hair was caught in the wind, and it looked so pretty. I thought to myself, *What a beautiful woman!* And then I realized, it was my wife!"

I love to purchase clothes during the off season. I used to do fashion shows for Gary. After dinner while he was relaxing, I would model all my new clothes. As I tried on each outfit, his eyes devoured me. No matter how many times I did these fashion shows, he'd say the same thing.

"You are so beautiful."

I'd laugh. "You are just saying that because I'm your wife."

"No, I'm saying it because it is the truth."

When it was time to purchase a greeting card for someone, Gary and I would spend an hour looking through all the cards. Early on in our relationship, I veered off and looked for a loving card for him. He read it, thanked me, and then veered off to find a loving card for me. We did this for nearly an hour, changing it up and finding a funny card for each other. We laughed afterwards and he said, "Well, that solves our card giving for a year." We continued that tradition throughout our marriage.

May 2018

Most assisted living facilities are not locked down, but the one Gary found was. It was one level, and all exterior doors had a keypad requiring a code to unlock. As the disease progressed, Gary might wander. I would not have to worry about him walking out. When Gary's mobility declined, he would not need to take stairs. Nor would he need cognition to use an elevator between floors. I felt certain that he would be able to stay as his disease progressed. At least that was the plan.

The facility was new, and the rooms were large. When Gary arrived there were ten residents, but the facility could accommodate up to fifty. Most rooms could accommodate a bed, a set of nightstands, couch, coffee table, mini fridge, and dresser, and there was a hook-up for cable TV and a landline. Wi-Fi was also available. Each room was furnished with an armoire and a twin bed. There were adequate shelves and laminated floors. The windows were large, which brightened the room. Attached to the room was a large bathroom with walk-in shower, handrails, and a shower seat. There was also a toilet, sink, and lots of shelves to store things.

Residents enjoyed three hot meals a day with snacks and drinks in the mid-afternoon. The activity director planned events for the residents such as manicures, pedicures, bingo, arts and crafts, and outdoor excursions such as leaf peeping (viewing fall foliage) and fishing. They also brought bands and singers in. Gary had his car parked outside his room. He could still drive, and he could come and go as often as he pleased.

There was a resident van that could transport residents to appointments depending on the van's schedule. Visitors were welcome at any time and encouraged to join in during special events like Fourth of July 4 picnics, Thanksgiving and Christmas dinners, and movie nights. Rockers lined the porch, and a huge, fenced courtyard offered the residents and their dogs a place to congregate and socialize. The facility provided medication management and assistance with daily activities. It also assisted with feeding if necessary and offered special accommodation for those in a wheelchair or requiring oxygen. A resident was turned away if they required IVs or feeding tubes. The primary doctor was offsite but visited the facility monthly, as did a hairstylist. All laundry and cleaning services were provided daily. A podiatrist, physical therapist, palliative care consultant, or hospice provider needed to be referred and brought in. There was an administrator and care manager available 24/7. Their phone numbers were both programmed into my phone. Cost? $3,200 a month.

This is inexpensive compared to what is available in other states. Most assisted living facilities nationwide average $5,000 a month ($7,000 for memory care). However, costs for memory care can go as high as $14,000 a month. Often the price does not include Depends, hairstylists, medication management, cable TV, landline phone, private nurses, or in-home sitters, which are often required. Prices will go up as healthcare needs rise. Some facilities charge a community fee totaling $1,000 or the cost of the first month's rent. Facilities are not covered under Medicare.

In-home care is even more expensive. It averages $35 an hour. At this rate, a fifty-six-hour week will cost $280 per day, $1,960 per week, and an average $7,840 a month—all out of pocket. For many caregivers, this is not nearly enough: many dementia patients require 24/7 supervision, which raises the cost astronomically. Interviewing candidates, managing caregivers, and ensuring competence (background checks and training in dementia) are extremely time-consuming tasks. Many caregivers install cameras so they can monitor what is happening in their home. This is also time-consuming.

Gary was very pleased to be moving. He knew he needed a safety net, and assisted living would provide it and allow him to retain his independence longer. He would be much closer to town and would be around people rather than isolated in our mountain home. I felt no guilt, as I firmly believed it would provide the care and attention that Gary needed. During the day, he could visit my dad or sister-in-law. It was on my way home from work, so I could drop by daily, and we could enjoy time out on weekends. I wanted to spend as much time as I could with him while he still had life left in him and provide some level of joy in the last chapter of his life.

I compiled a list of things that I needed to buy for Gary's new home. I decided to purchase bedding, drapes, a bathroom set, wall pictures, wall clock, mini refrigerator, and a TV for his room. Because the room at the facility was quite large, I made half of it a sitting area. That is where I put his TV, two end tables with lamps, a coffee table, his mini refrigerator, and a sofa. The other half of the room would house his bed, dresser, and armoire, which the facility provided. I wasn't concerned about the twin bed, as Gary was accustomed to a twin bed at our former home. When it was set up it resembled a studio apartment.

The one stipulation Gary had was his dog.

"I want my dog with me. If he can't come with me, I don't want to live there."

The facility allowed residents to have a dog, so Chase was readily accepted, even though he was a much larger dog than they normally allowed. Chase was a mixed lab weighing about 75 pounds.

Gary had an end room, which overlooked the parking lot and was right down the hall from the fenced courtyard that Chase would love. I knew Chase would be happy spending time in the yard with Gary and the other resident dogs.

Gary and I met with an attorney and reviewed Gary's POAs, living will, and advanced directives. The attorney asked Gary if he wanted revisions to his existing will. Before any paperwork was signed, the attorney gave him a mental assessment. Should anyone question Gary's intent, he would be able to testify in court that Gary was of sound mind. Gary and I also met with his physician and got a signed DNR (do not resuscitate) form.

As Gary and I were exiting the attorney's office, he asked Gary to wait in the lobby for a few minutes. He explained he wanted to speak with me.

Once Gary exited the room, I asked, "What's up? Is there a problem?"

"No, no problem. I just want you to know, Rose, that you can get a court-appointed guardian for Gary. They would handle his insurance payments and make sure he had an allowance and other things that he needs."

"Why would I do that?" I questioned.

"Well, Rose, you are not obligated in any way to watch over Gary. It would take you out of the picture, and the guardian would make sure his needs were taken care of. You can go forward with your life."

"Huh? I would never abandon Gary. He'd have no one to provide love or compassion. Plus, who would take him on outings? Visit him or buy him goodies? Who would be there during hospitalizations? Take him to the doctor's appointments? Advocate for him? I could never do that! I promised Gary I'd never abandon him. So far neither son has volunteered to look after their father." I was totally caught off-guard by what he was saying. I now had the support of a facility that would help me. I didn't know that the safety net would develop a lot of holes over the years, but assisted living remained a good decision. I wasn't taking on the full responsibility of care, as I would be if we were living together.

"I understand," he replied, "But I've had many clients do this journey. It gets rough. Very rough. If you change your mind, it's an option. Even with Gary in a facility it's going to be very hard. I've witnessed this firsthand."

"Thank you," I said. "That's not an option I'd ever take. I love Gary too much to let him do this journey alone."

Move Day

Gary decided to make the move before our home sold. I tried to convince him to wait, but he wanted to be closer to town. I sensed he was fearful of being alone in the mountain home all day while I worked. And I'm sure he got anxious driving our mountain road to the highway.

Gary wasn't at all anxious about the move, but sadness had lingered in me every day since his diagnosis. I told Gary there was no rush. "The house is not sold yet! I'll hire someone to look after you while I'm at work." But Gary was adamant. "I'll be closer to town; I'll be with people, and I'll have Chase with me. It's going to be okay." Even though I knew it was the right thing to do, without family support in that decision, I felt a sense of guilt and trepidation.

This stage of dementia was very difficult to comprehend, even for someone up front and personal with it. Most of the time Gary walked around in a state of total confusion. Other times, like in the discussion about when to move or with the attorney, he had clarity. At times even his articulation was good. He still looked youthful and healthy, so his appearance gave no indication of his diagnosis. Sometimes in the dark of night I thought, *could the neuropsychologist be wrong?* But then I reminded myself that his long-term insurance would not cover long-term care if they had not assessed him and determined he needed help with his daily living activities.

After receiving no offer of help from any family member with the transition, I called a neighbor and asked if he could move some furniture into Gary's room. I was ashamed to ask, but I had no choice. *Wouldn't this person wonder why someone from our family was not helping?*

I carried the emotional and physical task of moving Gary into assisted living alone. *Is family normally absent when a loved one is moved into a facility? Isn't that a major life event that they would want to be part of? Someone? Anyone?* It is emotionally difficult for someone to transition their loved one into assisted living, memory care, or a nursing facility. It carries undeserved guilt, loss, and memories of what was.

I had barely digested the fact that Gary had dementia, and now I was facing this. I thanked God that my heart was large, but I struggled for an answer that would satisfy me as to how family could disconnect from Gary and me so easily.

When I arrived at the facility, all the furniture was moved in. I spent a good part of the day arranging things. I wanted to make it as comfy and cozy as possible and make sure that Gary had everything he needed. Gary was happy that day and went down to the dining hall to enjoy his first meal. I opted out of going. I was struggling with a plate full of emotions, and I had no appetite for anything else.

While Gary was out of the room, I collapsed on his sofa. The physical work wasn't exhausting, but my emotions were spent. The administrator entered the room with more papers to sign, and I started to cry. Every emotion I had been holding in so that I would have a brave face for Gary escaped. My mind kept regurgitating the thought, *this cannot be happening!*

The administrator understood and sat beside me. She reached her arm around me. I searched for every ounce of willpower to pull myself together. I wanted to wake up from the nightmare I was living. My mind was questioning the reality of the situation. *Gary has dementia? Gary is now in an assisted living facility? But he's only 76! A very young 76! He's so healthy.*

After I pulled myself together, I walked down to the dining hall. Gary was at the table finishing his meal. He did not appear upset. I began crying again as soon as I reached my car. I would be spending the night without my husband or my dog. The marriage I knew was truly over.

No one called to ask, *how did the transition go?*

Ralph

Gary's son and I had a good relationship after his parents divorced. He was fourteen at the time. Gary was able to spend every weekend with him, and occasionally I would join them. I felt he and his father shared a good relationship. Gary helped him rebuild a car, they went on hunting trips together, and they always seemed to enjoy each other's company. I never heard them argue.

There was a twelve-year age difference between him and me and a twelve-year age difference between his dad and me. Throughout his son's teenage years and early adulthood, we often spent time together, and many times we double dated and shared a vacation. My heart readily accepted him as my stepson. Gary and I did not marry until Ralph was twenty.

His son moved a state away, got married, and had two beautiful daughters. We shared as much time as we could at their birthdays, picnics, and holidays. Each event was filled with laughter and fun. There was never any conflict or discord. When we moved to North Carolina in 2000, Ralph was thirty-four years old. He was extremely busy with his career and had made a beautiful home for his family. Gary and I were proud of his accomplishments.

Gary and I longed to get out of the snow and ice, so when he was offered an early retirement package, he grabbed it. When we relocated, we had planned to visit up North at least twice a year, but it became impossible. So much for planning. Still, we managed annual visits to visit my sister's family and his son's family. Gary and Ralph spoke by phone throughout the year. Both had busy schedules. I did my best to keep in touch with my daughter-in-law and the grandkids, but it's never quite the same as when you live closer. We were all busy with careers and raising children, and time was limited.

Steve

1994

I was relaxing in the middle of May, healing from a broken leg. I let my mind drift and began remembering three years prior, when Gary and I had attended preadoption workshops. As enthused as we were to adopt, our excitement did not last. My career, travel, and freedom quickly returned to center stage. I told myself, if the Lord wants me to have a child, he will bring him to me.

It was not that I could not bear a child of my own. I just did not relish the idea of staying home to care for an infant, and I felt it was foolish to have a baby and use daycare. But I loved children. Gary and I agreed. Why not provide a home for a child who had none? I had no doubt that I could love an adopted child as my own.

I was forty years old, and I knew that if I was going to adopt a child it should be soon. As I sat there musing, something came over me, and I said out loud, "Well, St. Jude, I am forty years old. If you want me to adopt a child, you better make it soon because I am getting old." It was then that I heard the phone ring.

I remember starting to laugh. Speaking to no one in particular, I said, "that was quick." I grabbed my cane and made my way into the kitchen to answer the phone.

"Hello."

"Am I speaking to Mrs. Jordan?"

"This is she."

"This is Linda Smith from the Department of Social Services, and I'm wondering if you are still interested in adopting a child."

I stood there for a moment, caught between fear that someone was in my house and utter disbelief.

"Why are you calling me?"

"Well, Mrs. Jordan, we need a home for a seven-year-old boy, and I'm looking through my records. I see from the paperwork you filled out that age, gender, or race is not a factor in adopting a child."

"Yes, that's right. But that was three years ago!"

"Are you still interested in adopting?"

"I don't know. You caught me off guard. I must think about this. I haven't thought about adopting in three years! Would you mind calling me back tomorrow?"

She sounded desperate. "We really need a home for this child. He's been in the system for seven years, and he needs to leave his current foster home. It's through no fault of his own, but the foster mom cannot care for him any longer. He'll need to go into residential care, as we have no place for him to go."

My mind was racing. "I need to think. This is all very sudden. I'll have to talk to my husband. Call me back tomorrow!"

"Okay. Around this time? Is that okay?"

"Yes, that will be fine."

I hung up the phone and hobbled back to my chair. *Huh? Did that call just happen? No, it couldn't have. Adoption? Are you kidding me? I don't know. I don't know.*

But within a week of meeting Steve, Gary and I accepted the challenge of adopting a child. We let our hearts lead without giving any consideration to how it might affect our lives.

The Rest of 2018

Gary suffered a bout of dehydration, a banged-up knee, an unspecified rash, and a trip to the ER in his first six months of assisted living. The reason for a trip to the ER wound up being a case of indigestion. I was quickly learning that almost every medical concern at an assisted living facility requires a trip to the ER. Assisted living does not have onsite nurses or doctors.

Chase was also becoming a challenge. Despite four different harnesses, he kept pulling out of them. I thought it was because Chase was unhappy, but he only broke loose when he was in front of the facility. Homeless cats loved to hang out there. And like his namesake, Chase loved to chase. I was very mindful when I returned him to the facility to hold the leash tight. But Gary could not remember to do this. The staff wound up chasing after the dog if Gary decided to take him for a walk or when he returned home.

A nurse from the long-term insurance company and a memory care specialist both needed to assess Gary quarterly. These appointments were extremely painful to watch. Gary no longer remembered the current month, year, or season. When asked, "If there was a fire on the stove, what would you do?" he answered, "Turn off the stove."

Despite a prescription for memantine, which was supposed to help with language, he was having more difficulty finding words. He referred to the dog food as pebbles. When I asked, "Where's the pebbles?" he'd hand me a dog biscuit. I needed to measure out the dog food and treats and place them in labeled baggies. I taped instructions on his wall describing how and what time to feed the dog.

As each month passed, I saw more and more decline. I bought a Swiffer mop. Despite showing Gary how to secure the cloth to the bottom of the mop, he could not process or remember the task. He'd ask, "How do you do that again?"

I brought a laptop into his room and loaded it with memory games for first graders. He could perform the games if I sat beside him and instructed him. He enjoyed playing them. But once I left, he could not open the game or play it unsupervised. I put sticky notes with instructions on the keyboard, but he could not process the instructions. Every time I showed him how to get into and play the game, it appeared as if he was seeing it for the first time. He'd ask repeatedly, "How do you do that again?"

Determined to find something for him to do unassisted, I got him a deck of cards. He loved to play solitaire. However, I discovered he could no longer play. I tried teaching him how to use the cards as a match game. He could not match the cards.

Each visit I arrived with a new purchase. I tried coloring books, connect the dots, and easy puzzles—anything I could find for a typical first grader. I saw Gary grow more and more frustrated as he realized he could not do these things. Although his mood was upbeat, he often said, "I hope this doesn't get any worse." I just kept reassuring him that I would be there to help him.

Gary was still driving and decided to go for a visit to my sister-in-law. Halfway there he became concerned that he was too early and decided to go for a drive. He got lost and grew frightened. He began turning the car around in all directions until he finally recognized something. He was very distressed when he shared this. He had driven that road dozens of times before. Although he wore a lifeline alert around his neck, he could not remember to push the 911 button. I also noticed unexplained dents in his car and witnessed him run a red light. We had a memory care specialist appointment scheduled in December, and I made a mental note to share this with the doctor.

He had been going to Senior Life Solutions, a therapy group for seniors, three times a week for two years. He loved the people there, and it gave him a routine. However, by the time end of year rolled around, he was experiencing more and more difficulty processing what the attendees and facilitators were saying and/or doing. He announced he would no longer be attending.

At the memory care appointment in December, the specialist asked, "Do you regularly exercise?" Gary replied, "My dog walks me."

The doctor and I both noted his humor was still intact. He had gained thirteen pounds since entering assisted living, and we were pleased about that.

Before I had the opportunity to discuss the driving incident, the doctor discussed with Gary the results of tests he took that day. He explained that they revealed he had difficulty with visual-spatial and executive function tasks, which might affect his driving. He encouraged Gary to take a formal OT (occupational therapy) evaluation with CarePartners, who would do an assessment and provide recommendations related to his functional ability to drive.

The oral exam would cost $250, and the behind-the-wheel driving exam would add another $250. Gary accepted the recommendation, but his intense gaze and creased forehead registered worry. He said in a low voice to no one in particular, "My memory isn't as good as it used to be."

For Christmas I bought a phone for him. It had slots to insert photos of family members. I programmed everyone's number into speed dial. If he wanted to call my father, for instance, he would find the photo and press the number above it. When I asked Gary if he liked the phone, he asked, "Who are these people?" I pulled out all the photos and replaced them with names. Like other unexplained symptoms, he was able to recognize handwritten names but not photos.

I also gifted him a clock that digitally displayed the date and time and whether it was morning, afternoon, or evening. I programmed it to prompt him when it was time to eat breakfast, to have drinks throughout the day, and to go to bed.

It had only been six months since he transitioned to assisted living, but the decline was noticeable. I had absolutely no idea the challenges of this disease and the care it entailed. I was spending much more time at the facility and answering calls than I anticipated. The disease weighed on me like an anchor dragging me to the ocean floor. Most times I exited the facility I left in tears. *Am I as strong as I'll need to be?*

Gary's symptoms — mild/moderate dementia
End of 2018

- Apathetic.
- Flat affect almost all the time.
- Experienced no joy with people, things, life in general.
- Exhibited uncharacteristic behaviors like anger when he was confused.
- He lacked the social skills he once had, he barely interacted in a room full of people.
- He was unable to process instructions even if written down.
- He was starting to get anxious, not wanting to screw up.
- He lacked any skill set he once had (building, plumbing, mechanics, etc.)
- He was withdrawing more and more from life.
- Things he'd say:

  – I can't remember shit anymore.

  – Pretty soon I won't remember who I am.

  – I hope this doesn't get worse.

His heart knows me, and he always expresses gratitude.

Blind and ignorant to the challenges that lay ahead

My humanitarian trait leads the way

There had been other similar times in my life that I'd accepted a challenge without much forethought. I've always believed, if you *think* too much about doing something, it causes fear. Fear limits pursuing dreams, taking risks, and doing what is right. The devil loves when we succumb to our insecurities. I'm a person who believes there are no limits on what I can do. The most motivating words I can hear are, *you can't do that!* Please watch me.

If I had let my brain direct me on whether to care give Gary, I would have analyzed and researched all available information. The left side of my brain had served me well in life, when, for example, I worked as an IT specialist or completed a master's degree in one year instead of the standard two. With all the facts on hand I would not have agreed to do it.

But it's that heart of mine that wins the race against my brain every single time. I am built to accept any challenge, but everything we choose to do in life has consequences. Sometimes I grab the end of the rope and play tug of war with all the obstacles wanting to pull me down in the mud. A lot of the time that's where I land, face first. The chore of getting up despite being dirty tires me. But I get up! Because quitting is not part of my vocabulary.

The roller coaster ride begins

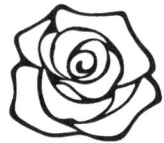

"I will do nothing lightly.
When I walk, I will walk heavily.
When I fight, I will fight with conviction.
When I speak, I will speak strongly.
When I feel, I will feel everything.
When I love, I will love with everything."

EVAN TANNER

January 22, 2019

Gary and I arrived at 10:30 a.m. at CarePartners for a driving evaluation. I decided that I would not wait in the waiting room, but I would attend the appointment with Gary to make sure he was given a fair shake. I was becoming very protective of Gary because of his limited capacity. I joked with him on the way to the test and reassured him that, whatever happened, we would deal with it together. I drove his car so that he could take the behind-the-wheel test in a familiar vehicle.

We were ushered into an evaluation room by an OT specialist. She was extremely polite and kind to Gary. She encouraged him to relax and told him not to worry if he did not get a perfect score. She would do everything she could to give him a restricted license. Gary was seventy-seven years old at the time and had been driving for sixty-one years. He looked at her and said, "Give me a gold star." I wanted to cry.

The OT specialist began by evaluating his upper extremity strength for vehicle requirements. There were no concerns. Next, his lower extremities were assessed (range of motion, strength, proprioception, sensation with socks and shoes off). Again, no concerns. He passed and got his gold star for standing/sitting and balance/mobility.

He was then given a set of pedals to measure his reaction time. He required a .75 reaction time to drive without restrictions, and he received a .76. The test proceeded. I thought, *Okay, he'll have a restricted license. We're still good.*

Gary wears eyeglasses, but no abnormalities were noted with head position, eye fatigue, or ptosis. However, the OT specialist noticed that Gary often closed his eyes during testing. I tried to tell him telepathically, *"Stop doing that!"* as I had told him numerous times. He had been prone to keep his eyes closed since 2015, when he had begun taking Keppra. When I questioned his neurologist about this, he insisted it was normal. I never understood how he could walk and not trip with his eyes half-mast.

A journey of love

It was very apparent as the testing proceeded that Gary was struggling. He was unable to look forward and be aware of stimuli in his right and left peripheral fields. He was easily distracted and had poor road sign knowledge. The Short Blessed Test yielded a score of eighteen. Impaired memory is proven with a score of eight or greater. Gary yielded a score of zero on the Clock Drawing Tests, which measure cognitive, motor, and perceptual skills. A score of four or less can be a predictor of unsafe driving.

In the final analysis Gary failed the test. The specialist recommended that he not go ahead with the behind-the-wheel evaluation. The depth of sadness on Garys face made me want to bolt out of the room. But I didn't. I could see the specialist's eyes radiating love through Gary's pain.

I'm an empath. I felt every fear, frustration, and inadequacy that Gary did. I wanted to turn those emotions off. I wanted to sit there as a stranger, a clinician, and have an *oh well, it is what it is* moment. But I was stuck in the sadness of his new reality.

"We will proceed with the road examination," I told the specialist. She offered a concerned look. I continued, "I'll pay the extra $250 to give Gary every possible opportunity to get a restricted license."

Gary walked to the testing vehicle. He appeared relieved that he had one last chance, but I knew he was also fearful. Gary was aware that his memory was impaired. If I were to read his mind, I imagined, I would hear him praying to the Lord to help him pass the test without screwing up. He was ahead of me, and I was grateful because I did not want his eyes to see the fear in mine. I did not know how failing the test would affect him. He had lost so much already.

I wondered at first why they weren't using Gary's car. *He'd be so much more familiar in his own vehicle.* But of course, I admonished myself. *They need to have control of the car. Just in case.* The vehicle he drove was dual controlled for safety.

Gary was able to walk to the car and open and close the door, put on his seatbelt, adjust the mirrors, seat, and steering wheel, and start

The roller coaster ride begins

the ignition. He appeared relaxed and ready to hit the road. *One more chance, babe, make it good.* My gut twisted, and I prayed Gary didn't see the fear on my face as I asked for the Lord's help.

I later learned that the test started well. Gary showed good lane maintenance, steering control, and speed regulation, and he was able to stop suddenly on two different occasions. He used his turn signals correctly seven out of eight times and navigated both traffic light and non-traffic light intersections.

The issues began when he was asked to change lanes. Over the course of two miles, he was unable to execute the command. He also hesitated when pulling into traffic. His multitasking skills were evaluated next. He was asked to find an Ingles supermarket, pull into the parking lot, and park. Gary drove past it. He was asked to look for speed limit signs, check his speedometer, and tell the test administrator the speed he was going. Most clients see at least 75 percent of signs. Gary saw only one out of seventeen.

We returned to the OT office, where staff recommended that Gary retire from driving and give up his license at the DMV. Some moments are unforgettable. I watched his face crumble along with his independence. He sat hunched in a defeated position with both hands resting on his lap. He did not lift his head, as he was unable to meet any of our eyes. And then he began sobbing as he had when he thought family was throwing him away. His entire body convulsed with the sorrow of a disease robbing him of his independence and self-sufficiency. It was just all too much. The shame, the embarrassment, and the loss of it all. I knew he felt like a complete failure.

I was glued to my chair, willing myself to become desensitized to my emotions. My tears would be of no help to Gary. I knew there was nothing I could say or do to ease his suffering. This was his experience, and somehow, in some way, he would need to accept it. I sat there questioning the Lord. Why had he chosen me to be Gary's caregiver? A job I felt totally inadequate for. *Why didn't you choose one of his sons, Lord? Will one of them call tonight and encourage their dad after this heart wrenching day? They both knew he was having his driving tested. Will anyone call who he supported and loved?* Gary had received very few calls since diagnosis, and no one was calling me to offer support or stay informed about Gary. I would occasionally receive a "How are you?" text, but there were few listening ears or offers of help.

I got up from my chair, gathered Gary's things, thanked the OT specialist, and said, "It's okay, babe. We got this." I hugged him as I ushered him to the car. "It's gonna be okay, it will. We'll figure this out."

I didn't want to pity myself. I never liked feeling pitiful; I liked having power and being strong. But I did waver between self-pity for myself and compassion for Gary many times during this journey. The self-pity came into play now, as I could not contemplate adding chauffeuring to my already jammed schedule. My body was exhausted from all the chores and to-do lists, plus my mind was already overwhelmed with emotions.

I cut this feeling short, put a smile on my face, and looped my arm into his. "You will be able to do everything without a car that you did with a car. I promise you, babe. I've got this." I said the words, but I was not at all sure how much more Gary or I could handle. My heart never hurt as much as it did that day. I was the only one consoling it.

One of the topics discussed on dementia support groups all the time is the difficulty of taking away a loved one's keys. It's very emotional for the driver because it's a symbol of autonomy, freedom, independence, and self-sufficiency. Why were Gary and I the only ones feeling this huge loss? I did not receive any calls afterward to ask, *how did the driving test go?* No one called Gary to empathize with the fact he had just lost a huge part of his independence. Was everyone desensitized to Gary's suffering? I wish I could have given immediate grace to those who appeared not to give a damm. But I did not possess the holy grail.

Over the next few months, family members made it clear they did not approve of *my* decision not to allow Gary to drive. Some said, "Everyone drives with dementia." Another said, "He can still drive on back roads!" When I offered that Gary would not feel good about running over a child because he could not stop in time, I was told I was being ridiculous and was taking away all his freedom. I was angry and annoyed at the insinuations that I was controlling Gary. I was protecting him and looking out for his best interests. It was easier for many to stay in denial than accept his disease, as I was forced to do. It was also easier to attack the caregiver than a disease they chose not to witness or be involved in.

Insinuations of being controlling follow caregivers on this journey all the time. I surmise it's because people who have chosen to stay away do not realize just how much the caregiver needs to do and how many decisions they must make to keep their loved ones safe. The truth was I took charge and protected Gary from symptoms he could not control. I protected him so that he didn't feel ashamed, uncomfortable, or scared. If anyone had control, it was the disease. I was just the one who had the strength to meet it head on. I realized then that many did not have a clue what we were dealing with. But I wasn't going to make it my job to educate or inform them. If they were interested, they could phone us or get involved.

Easter Weekend

I visited Gary on Good Friday. I treated him to his favorite chicken dinner at Bojangles before I returned him to the facility. On Saturday I called and asked if he would like to go to a movie. He didn't sound like himself when we spoke; he was almost robotic. But I dismissed the red flag and headed over to the facility. I phoned the care manager and told her to make sure he was ready and that I was on my way to pick him up.

While driving I received a call. It was the care manager. She had gone down to Gary's room and phoned to say, "He's not right, Rose. He seems very confused. More so than usual." I began to question her when she screamed, "OMG. I think he's having a stroke or something." I disconnected the call and calmed myself as I gave the car more gas.

When I entered his room, I saw Gary on the floor with a CNA cradling his head. He was having a grand mal seizure. The care manager had called EMS. I knew from experience that there was literally nothing to be done. When the EMS arrived, they checked his breathing, and I followed the ambulance to the hospital.

I had them do bloodwork to check his seizure medication level. I wanted to make sure that the facility did not mismanage his dose. Gary had been hospitalized for seizures in the past, so I knew they would begin administering more seizure medication. And that he would be admitted for a few days or up to a week for observation.

In the past, Gary would be calm and sedate after a seizure. However, his dementia was making him very antsy. He wanted to leave, and he remained agitated despite reassurances. The doctor ordered Ativan (a sedative), but that appeared to intensify his agitation. I phoned Ralph and told him I needed him. I hadn't had a break in a long time, and I felt unable to sit at Gary's bedside for eight-to-ten-hours until he was able to sleep. Hospital sitters are rarely available for dementia patients, so caregivers are expected to keep them calm, in bed, fed, and entertained. If a caregiver is not available, nurses will be given an order to sedate them with Haloperidol (an antipsychotic), which delays discharge and lingers in their system. I did not want that to happen.

Ralph shared that he was extremely busy with work but offered to come for three days. He arrived one day prior to discharge. I was out of work the entire week. I felt extremely uncomfortable when he entered the room. We had not communicated since his dad's diagnosis. We met in Gary's hospital room, and after pleasantries I invited him to dinner.

Not completely knowing what lay ahead, I explained that I was not looking for financial support or help in caring for his dad. I said, "Your father can stay where he is. I've established a good rapport with the staff, I make sure he has whatever supplies he needs, I visit him, take him on outings, and provide emotional support and love. But when your dad is hospitalized or the time comes when he needs more care, I need and expect cooperation from you. I encourage you to periodically check in with me and to call your dad. He needs the love of his family!"

"Why don't you ask Steve for help?" he asked.

I answered. "I don't hear from him. I've attempted but I've had trouble communicating with him about Dad. I cannot handle the additional stress. Give him a call if you feel he'll be receptive."

I entered this journey because of the love in my heart for Gary, but it had now been five years since my return to our marriage. I had mixed feelings on whether I could continue caregiving Gary without any family support or physical help during a crisis. The facility safety net I thought I could rely on did not extend to hospitalizations. I also struggled with the fact that our family appeared oblivious to the seriousness of the disease, the difficulty I had witnessing it, and the physical and emotional toll it was having on me. My anger and resentment were starting to build.

Flashback

Gary and I loved to travel. He and I both had a month vacation from our jobs, so we used it for new adventures and travel. We went on cruises; traveled to Las Vegas, Los Angeles, Lake Tahoe, San Francisco, Washington, DC, Laguna Beach, Disney World, Barbados, Hawaii, and Canada; and took road trips through the southern states, anywhere our hearts desired. One year he needed to go to Germany for business and offered, "Come with me. You'll have no trouble roaming around while I work. The second week I'll have off. We'll rent a car and travel the countryside."

It sounded like a great proposition, so off we went. We spent time with a German friend and his wife and had the pleasure of being taken to non-tourist areas. His friend passed me a language book so that I could attempt to communicate in their language when we went off on our own. I secretly hoped that it would not be necessary. My New Jersey accent intruded on every translation, making it more difficult for people to understand me.

We visited castles and quaint cities and experimented with the different foods the country had to offer. I closed my eyes as Gary drove the Autobahn. It was only when he drove that Gary's personality changed from meek and mild to a spirit consumed with speed and risk. The speed limit is 80 miles per hour, but drivers are allowed to drive faster in unrestricted areas. I kept my yelling in check as Gary practiced being a NASCAR driver.

Before we left, Gary insisted on purchasing German liverwurst for a friend. We had some difficulty finding a deli but walked into a store offering cheese and lunchmeats. As other patrons were being served, I got out my language book and practiced asking for a pound of liverwurst. When it came my turn, I gave it my best shot. No luck. The server looked at me like I had two heads. I attempted a couple more times before I looked at Gary and said, "Forget it. I don't see any liverwurst in the display case. Let's just leave." We had everyone in the place looking at us as they waited for their turn.

Suddenly Gary started pounding on his chest. *Huh?*

"What are you doing?" I asked. "You look silly."

Then I heard him say as he continued to pummel his chest, "Leber! Leber!" And I realized *Oh my God, he's attempting to communicate liver.* By this point I was laughing hysterically, and I was convinced we would be thrown out of the place or that EMS would be called.

Suddenly the server threw up her hands and said, "Aww, Leberwurst! Leberwurst!" I backed out of the store because I was in a very giddy mood and could not stop the laughter or the tears cascading down my face. I feared if I did not exit quickly, I'd feel traces of pee running down my legs.

Gary came out shortly afterwards carrying a few pounds of leberwurst and a huge smile. I looked at him and said, "You are a nut. You do know that, right? You almost made me pee my pants."

He began to laugh, "I got the liverwurst, didn't I?"

Sadly, by the time we got to the States, his leberwurst was rancid.

May 2019

The Last Home Visit

I decided to pick Gary up and take him to our mountain home. I was curious if he'd remember it. He had been at assisted living for a year. As I pulled off the highway and started up the seven-mile stretch to our home, I wondered whether Gary would remember anything.

"Babe, do you know where we are going?"

"I forget where you told me." He replied.

"I'm taking you to our home. The one you helped build. Do you remember this road?"

"No."

I was a bit surprised, but surely when we pulled into our driveway he would remember. After stopping the car in front of our garage, I let the dog out, and he raced to the ridge he was familiar with. He would look for his friends Maggie and Gunner. Gary exited the car and got very upset.

He shouted and clapped his hands. "Chase, come back!"

"Calm down. It's okay, babe. Chase will be back. He knows this area."

"No, he'll run away!" he said, very agitated.

"I promise you, babe, it's okay. Please, trust me. This used to be his home. He'll come back."

I led him to the front of the home. Pointing to the fence, I said, "You put that fence up, babe."

"I did? Where's Chase?"

"Chase will be back in ten minutes. I promise. Look over here at the foundation. You stoned that foundation, all by yourself. We hauled the stones up here by from Nantahala Gorge."

He looked surprised. I said nothing else as I led him into the home we built. As he entered the great room he said, "You have a very nice home."

I could feel tears forming. I forced them away. I walked him toward our bedroom. "This was our bedroom, babe." No recognition registered.

"It's nice," he replied.

I led him through the rest of the house. "See up there," I said pointing to the balcony. "That's where you sat on your computer. "There's two bedrooms and a bath up there."

"You have a big house," he said.

"Do you want to sit on the back porch?"

"No," he replied. "We should be heading back. We must find Chase."

As if on cue, Chase was waiting at the garage door. Gary was very happy to see him. I drove down the mountain not comprehending how Gary could not remember a house we put our hearts and souls into building. Such a brief period had passed! I reached for his hand and held it the rest of the way down.

I remembered what Harry, the regional ombudsman, had said to me, "Gary will remember little else but the room he stays in." But it was still difficult for my heart not to feel injured that our dream home no longer held any importance to Gary. He never asked to go back to it.

Very often people with dementia will say "I want to go home." When they say this, they will usually be in their home. The home they refer to is a state of mind, not a physical place. What they are trying to articulate is the desire to return to how they were, or the way things were. Or they are remembering their childhood home or a place where they felt whole, happy, and loved by people they are no longer able to identify. Dementia caregivers often rush to bring their loved ones back to their home from a facility, and as soon as they arrive, their loved ones will continue to say, "I want to go home. This isn't my home!"

Sister and brother-in-law visit Gary

My sister and her husband knew Gary before I did. They introduced us. They both loved him very much. On their annual trips to my dad's, they would make the time to visit Gary. I knew he was grateful for those visits, and so was I. Throughout the year, my sister and niece would send Gary cards and gifts, and they phoned him regularly.

When my sister visited, I was told, "meet us at the facility." I usually chose not to. The facility was my second home but not my happy place. I would not be able to share my heart on their visits with Gary. Their focus was on him, not me. I would not receive the attention I craved or their empathetic ear.

The few times I did go, I immediately saw the heart connection between Gary and them. I witnessed the same when Ralph visited. The smile, the chuckle, the glint in Garys eye told me that in that limited time he basked in the love his heart felt.

As soon as they were gone, Gary did not remember my sister or her husband. Not by name, not by a photograph, and not by a memory I shared with him. They needed to be present for his heart to feel the connection and know them.

Gary needed to be in what he now considered his home, his safe place, to feel comfortable visiting people. If he left the facility, he would feel secure only if I was with him. If visitors took him into another environment without me, he would have a hard time readjusting back home. The stress from that brief time away caused him undue anxiety. I'd get frequent calls from the facility describing how difficult it was for him when he returned home. The staff encouraged me to talk to visitors about keeping him onsite.

I encouraged the few visitors he had to stay inside the facility, but they felt I was being controlling and manipulative. They had not learned what I had. That what we feel is right for our loved one isn't always in their best interest. With dementia, it's important to always focus on the patient's reality, not how we perceive it.

July 2019

To say I was overwhelmed with happiness would be an understatement. Our large mountain home that had been on and off the market since 2006 was under contract. The sale would not make me wealthy; the housing crisis had depreciated the home. However, to be free of the burden of its upkeep and mortgage was tremendous. In addition, I could now move into a more populated area. The isolation at the mountain home was affecting my mental health.

I contacted a realtor friend in Asheville, where I wanted to move. The first week out with her, I found the perfect town house. It was new, within my price range, and would accommodate most of my furniture. I was thrilled that I had found a new home so quickly. Even though it was an hour and a half from Gary, I would make it work.

The inspection of my home yielded a laundry list of items, but after careful review there was nothing major, and certainly nothing that would deter a sale. Finally, something was happening in my favor, and the burden of upkeeping this large home would be over.

Three weeks into the contract I received a call. It was from my realtor informing me the prospective owners had changed their minds. I was in utter shock that after waiting 13 years for a contract, it fell apart. When I regained my composure, my relationship with the Lord intensified. I told HIM, "*You want me here? Fine. I'll learn to accept that. I don't like it, but I'm not fighting it anymore. When you are ready, I'll be ready.*" I meant every word. I could not handle the stress of trying to sell this home another day.

August 2019

I felt my emotional and physical health deteriorating. By now I was consumed with anger and resentment because of the disconnect and lack of empathy or support from family. And I had a hard time removing myself from the sadness of dementia and Gary's suffering. I was exhausted from the additional chores of getting supplies, making visits, fielding facility calls, navigating an inadequate healthcare system, and chauffeuring Gary. Physically I found the stamina to do what needed to be done despite the tiredness. But it was getting harder to convince myself I could survive in the isolated world of caregiving.

Since I was a teenager, I had needed control over my life. I did not want to be tamed. I wanted to make my own choice as to how to live my life. Now I found myself without the freedom to do what I wanted when I wanted. I felt like a horse pulling a wagon filled with Gary's needs, with no room left for my own. It felt uncomfortable living for two when only one was getting the love and attention they needed to survive.

To find some inner peace, I bought a pair of sneakers and began to walk. Every morning I'd bound out of bed and pound the pavement for four miles. I not only found a more peaceful mind on those walks, but I also formed a relationship with the Lord that carried me through challenges that imprisoned me. I listened to Joyce Meyers on my cell phone and learned the word of God. I began feeling stronger and more empowered.

I grew up believing that our fate was in the Lord's hands. That he alone decides who we will be and what we will have. If we will be healthy or suffer from a disease. I didn't believe that anymore. I didn't believe that the Lord created disease. Gary was a good man and a good Christian. The Lord did not give him dementia. The Lord is not cruel. Regardless of what we choose to do, regardless of what happens in our lives, God is with us. Beyond a shadow of a doubt, I began to feel his true presence. He was steadfast, and from that point forward he never left the room.

Since a child, I had been the type of Christian that attended church because my parents told me if I didn't that I'd be destined to hell. I often sat through Mass with thoughts of being elsewhere and would glance at the clock counting the minutes until it was over.

I believed in the Lord, but my belief was limited to when I needed or wanted something. I would recite the prayers I learned in childhood and then hope that they were answered. Sometimes I'd even spend a dollar and light a candle in church. If the Lord didn't answer my prayers, I did not stop believing. I would just wait until the next time I needed or wanted something, and I'd repeat the process.

Gary's journey with dementia changed my belief in ways I didn't think possible. I became friends with the Lord. I sought him out when no one else was there. I'd whisper into the darkness, "All I have is God." I quickly changed that to, "I'm so thankful I have God."

October 2019

A dementia diagnosis does not mean that other life challenges stop for the caregiver. I had other responsibilities on my plate. One of them was watching over my dad. I noticed on a visit that he did not look well. He was ninety-four years old, and, although self-sufficient, his age dictated attention. When I mentioned my concern, he complained that since starting a new medication for his racing heart he could barely get off the couch. I scheduled a visit with his cardiologist. Dad was also complaining of shoulder pain. So, I scheduled an appointment with an orthopedic doctor. I felt guilty that my time with him was so limited, but I gave what time I had left.

The calls were coming in more often from assisted living, and my stress was increasing with the number of commitments I was shouldering. I needed to decide what I could eliminate from my plate. It couldn't be Gary. Or my dad. I still had all the responsibilities of handling life and home. It had to be my job. I'd lose my income, but I was lucky. I could still make my bills without that check.

My current job was doing behavior intervention and tutoring higher risk children and older youth. It was a happy job. No stress, just sheer enjoyment. I was semiretired and took the job strictly to help those who were struggling. It was very unlike the social work I had done in the past. Working in child welfare was almost as sad as caregiving Gary. But I loved teaching, and I loved children, so I grabbed the job when it was offered. The school community was like family to me, and I embraced every challenge and every group of children they sent me. It was my happy escape from the sadness of dementia.

A dementia caregiver provides an easier path to a death sentence. Patients don't give feedback or provide conversation or laughter. Rarely can they put a smile on your face. It's giving to another when all hope has been lost.

Working with youth to help them have a better life brings a different type of reward. The children I worked with provided me dozens of hugs a day, smiles, and laughter. They brought me back to happier, more carefree times. A time when the greatest gift was a lollipop, set of pencils, or something from a teacher's treasure chest.

I needed to give up the life preserver that took me away from dementia and provided countless hours of joy. I would miss these children terribly, and I knew they'd miss me too. I submitted my resignation to the school.

November 2019

Gary's birthday was November 19. A family member visiting from out of state asked me to bring Gary to my father's for birthday cake. I discussed it with Gary and told him I would not be going. It was stressful for me to be around family who I felt were neglecting and ignoring us.

"I don't know those people. I don't want to go," he shared. While his heart still held love for family, he no longer recognized many by face or name. He rarely saw the people who would be there. His anxiety was increasing daily.

I explained to him, "This is your family, you might have fun."

But he was adamant. "I do not want to go!" I reassured him that I would talk to them and make them understand.

"His feelings need to be respected. He has a right to make his own decision," I explained to family.

But they pushed, "We are his family! You shouldn't keep him from us. Dad wants him to be there."

I repeated that we needed to respect Gary's wishes. I said, "I asked him a few times, but got the same reply. He feels uncomfortable leaving his safe zone. He has little else left but to make his own decision on where he wants to go. Bring the cake to the facility. They have a huge room you can congregate in, and the staff will welcome you."

I thought that matter was settled until I phoned Gary that evening. When he didn't answer the phone, I called the main desk. I was told that his family had picked him up. I was very distraught that Gary's decision was ignored and my plea was dismissed. I felt like I had let him down. He was counting on me to communicate his feelings.

When I phoned Gary later, I asked what happened.

He communicated, "I didn't know what to say when they showed up. I didn't want to go, but I was afraid I'd hurt feelings."

I explained to him how sorry I was that it happened. "But you had a good time, right? They are your family. They just wanted to spend time with you."

"I didn't know any of the people. I just sat there. I told them I wanted to go, but they told me to wait a while. They said we were going to have cake. I just wanted to go home."

When I tried to explain to my family how hurt I felt that they had not listened to my pleas, I was told, "You are being silly. We are his family. He had a great time!" I know they meant no harm, but it's so important that the patient and caregiver's wishes be respected.

December 2019

Each week throughout the year, I methodically measured out dry dog food for Chase and placed it into marked baggies. Each baggie had the date with either a.m. or p.m. marked on it. In addition, I'd put wet food in containers marked Monday through Sunday. I wanted Gary to be able to feed our dog while he was still able.

On a visit, I noticed that Gary was overfeeding the dog. Two weeks of food disappeared in one week. I ordered an automatic dog feeder and water dispenser. Gary was also giving too many treats to the dog. So, I placed them in bags marked Monday through Sunday and gave them to the care manager with instructions. *The assisted living facility where he resided overextended themselves to keep Gary and Chase together and happy.*

Gary noticed the change and began to feel bad about himself.

"What is wrong with me? I can't do anything right! I can't even feed my dog." He looked so defeated and disgusted.

"It's okay, sweetheart. We have this. Let me help you. There's no reason for you to stress over Chase's food anymore. Won't it feel good that you won't have to worry about feeding him properly?"

"Yeah, I guess so."

"Okay, then. Let's not think about this anymore. You still have Chase with you, and he'll stay healthy because he won't be overeating. It's a win-win situation."

Gary had a nurse assessment required by his long-term insurance the next day. After painfully watching him struggle to answer the questions during the assessment, I told him to return to his room and that I'd be right there. Once out of hearing range, I turned to the nurse. "Is this necessary? It's not going to get better. These assessments are difficult for him, and it's hard for me to watch." I saw tears in the nurse's eyes. He wrote a note. The insurance company never requested another assessment.

The year finished with a tremendous windstorm. A large pine fell on the front of our mountain home. Thankfully, there was no major damage done to the home, but it cost $5,000 to have it removed. Home insurance covered a small part of it. *Despite dementia, caregivers have other stressors that need to be dealt with.*

Gary's symptoms — end of 2019
Moderate dementia

- Repeating, repeating, repeating.
- He could no longer make his bed.
- He needed help with buttoning shirts. "My fingers don't work anymore."
- He did not remember when he last ate.
- He could no longer pump gas.
- He needed help cutting his food.
- He could no longer fix his plate.
- He could no longer process a movie.
- He could no longer pull money from an ATM.
- His ability to read and process was greatly diminished.
- He could no longer feed the dog properly.
- He could no longer tell the time or differentiate between morning, afternoon, or evening.
- He no longer recognized family photographs.
- He did not know how to insert a CD into a CD player.
- He could not comb his dog.
- He changed clothes multiple times throughout the day.
- He needed help showering, shaving, and dressing appropriately.

- His anxiety was increasing. A friend would pick him up for church on Sundays. He would pace the hallways two and a half hours before his ride would arrive.

- He got very apprehensive when in the car. "Where are we going? This is so far! When am I going home?"

- As Gary watched me drive, he'd appeared shocked, "You really know how to get around!"

- The blinds in his room needed to always remain closed. He was fearful that someone could see in or that the rain and cold would come through his window.

His heart knew me, and he always expressed gratitude.

Where was I in this challenge of a dementia caregiver?

I started the journey not wanting to abandon another human. And yet it is I who now felt abandoned or ignored by family. My vision of what the journey would look like was vastly different from the reality I was experiencing. At the onset of Gary's diagnosis, I felt certain he would receive calls, empathy, support, and more visits from the family. After all, he was on borrowed time. I felt I would be blessed with listening and empathetic ears, encouragement, visits, and an occasional helping hand without having to ask. Gary and I had supported many people in our life. I felt it would be reciprocal. But so far that vision was just a vision. The reality was an eye-opener, and a sad one at that. My heart, which had led me to the challenge of being a caregiver, felt broken. My ignorance of the disease and all it entailed was becoming more and more obvious.

I felt stuck between a rock and a hard place. I felt the value system that had brought me to this point was wearing thin as emotional and physical exhaustion set in. Two years had passed since Gary's diagnosis, and the aloneness was saturating every cell of my being. I was not comfortable accepting the disconnect from others. I spent hours and days trying to analyze and process our family's motives for not calling, offering support, or visiting.

Hurt is more saturating than anger. Anger is just a symptom of a much larger feeling. It tends to happen quickly, explode, and then dissipate. Hurt lingers in dark crevices of the mind and is usually visited by a therapist. It's like a skin cancer that if left untreated festers and grows. How does one nurse hurt? I had no idea, so I shoved it into the far corners of my brain. I had more important work to do than to regurgitate it daily. But when it resurfaced, it had gained strength.

Many times, I'd get a three-word text from a family member. *How ya doing?* Or *how's Gary doing?* I'd struggle to answer. Do I just say, "Okay," meaning we're still alive? Or do I sit and write chapters of all that was happening in his life and mine? If they were really interested, wouldn't they pick up the phone?

If I got that rare phone call from family and began unloading, I'd get interrupted with advice and/or criticism on what I needed to do. When I said to someone, "Just listen to me!" I was told, "If you don't want my input, then you should talk to a wall. Communication is a two-way street."

I had difficulty comprehending how anyone could offer advice on a situation they were not part of. I was in this marathon; I wasn't a runner who showed up at a checkpoint. Plus, I had a master's in clinical social work. I spent a good deal of my life helping others, finding resources, investigating all the possibilities of advocacy, and working in a person's best interest. It boggled my mind that some appeared ignorant of this fact. Sometimes I felt blessed to be ignored. It saved me the hurt of having to regurgitate Gary's illness over and over, being misunderstood, or being told my actions were wrong. Other times I felt cursed by the lack of caring, understanding, and isolation the disease brought to my door.

When I gave hurt the time, I examined it. What was it I was feeling? The answer came quickly. I felt emotionally neglected by the people who purported to love me. I can't give an answer for how Gary was feeling because dementia was playing so many tricks on his brain. But when he would look at me and say, "I want to find my people," I believe what he was trying to articulate was *his need to feel the love of the people who were once in his life.* Although Gary's executive functioning was haywire, his heart was intact. He didn't recognize names or faces or know how he was related to them, but his heart always held love.

It was not my job to get our family to participate. From the few that called, any suggestion to visit was met with reasons or excuses why they could not. Busyness was a common theme. And yet these same people found time for family vacations and events. Evidence was on Facebook. Shouldn't a loved one's death sentence trump a busy schedule? Gary's dementia was on a timeline. Another excuse was, *don't guilt me.* That clearly was not the intention when I suggested a visit. I knew the clock was ticking, and Gary was losing ground. He could not articulate his need, so I felt I needed to be his voice. I did not want him to exit the world feeling unloved. Most of the time, our family's absence was accompanied by silence. Family members became ghosts. I wanted Gary to feel the arms of the family he loved. I wanted them to tell him how much they loved him. I wanted him to have a chance to say goodbye. *Was that a bad thing?*

When I spoke about abandonment, one family member suggested, "Maybe you never had them." I wasn't sure how to respond other than, "Guess they had me fooled." I'm certain that if Gary had not received a dementia diagnosis, we would both be exactly where we left off with visits, calls, and feelings of belonging. Perhaps now with the self-awareness of where we stood, I'd never walk again in an imaginary universe. I'd never have a reason to feel joined to them.

Truth be told, if they came, and Gary's heart enjoyed them, he'd forget the visit ten minutes after they left. But he'd have those ten minutes. And I always hoped that when they visited, they would share time with me too. My heart did not forget the memory of them.

I asked Gary once, "Are you sad?"

"Not anymore," he replied. I felt his sadness had turned into acceptance. And with acceptance, loss of hope. His response brought such mourning. I thought about the long, lonely hours he spent in a world he no longer knew. *Did anyone else spend time thinking of this?*

I am not the kind of person to hold my tongue. Although sometimes it spoke in bitterness, it usually did not. I am human and not perfect. My voice sought understanding, compassion, and empathy. It spoke facts about the situation and the hurt I was feeling by the actions of our family. People often don't want to hear the truth if they think their character or ones they love are being questioned. I get that. Self-examination is hard.

One person who offered help did so based on their convenience, not my need or Gary's best interest. When I'd turn it down or attempt to explain why it would not be helpful, I was told, "Nothing I offer is right with you." If I suggested what would be more helpful, it was denied. I internalized this rejection and felt as if I had done something wrong. That made it more difficult for me to ask for help.

Family abandonment is a common theme on the dementia journey. Online dementia support groups testify to it every single day. Reading so many online posts helped me not to personalize it. However, I often thought, if a man like Gary, who never had a conflict with anyone and who loved and supported people his whole life, was forgotten, what chance did someone like me have?

When I shared with a family member, "I've been abandoned!" The reply was, "No you haven't!" With emotional abandonment, one feels left behind or discarded. It causes emotional pain and anxiety. When someone is physically abandoned, support or help is withdrawn. So yes, given these definitions, I felt that Gary and I were emotionally and physically abandoned by most family members.

The caregiver not only feels hurt for themselves, but they also feel it for the person with dementia. I always felt more hurt for Gary's abandonment than for my own. I was not the one losing my mind. I was not the one on borrowed time. In my mind, those facts made abandoning him worse.

A lot of caregivers lose not only family but also friends. I did not. My friends supported me throughout my journey. Sadly, most lived out of state. They had good listening ears and offered to fly out, but I didn't want to burden them. Plus, it wouldn't be helpful for Gary, about whom I was most concerned.

Like dementia, which is totally unpredictable and makes no sense, so are people's attitudes toward the patient and caregiver. A million-dollar question is *why is it so prevalent on a dementia journey that patients and caregivers are abandoned and/or ignored?* I could list reasons offered on support groups such as busyness, I want to remember them as they were, they won't know I'm there anyway, or I can't handle that kind of stuff. But I'll accept the challenge and offer other thoughts or possible reasons.

I feel being sensitive to another's suffering and needs is a human trait. Some people don't have that telescopic ability to extend their sensitivity past themselves and their immediate family. Or perhaps some, rather than face the reality of this disease, will bring up relational issues to keep them at a safe distance. A third reason might be that some view dementia as a mental illness which is stigmatized rather than a brain condition. Dementia is usually associated with mental illness due to symptoms of anxiety, depression, apathy, and strange behaviors. I needed to find a way to accept that not everyone was like me or walk around with a shoulder of hurt for not one but two people.

Other million-dollar questions. Is a caregiver supposed to forget all the absences when the journey is over? Pick up where they left off? Are reconnections even possible? I understood forgiveness, but how does one forget? The people you felt you knew going into the journey are not the same people you know when you exit. Did everyone get a free pass after Gary was buried? The answers to these questions haunted me daily.

Pandemic

"Sorrow looks back, Worry looks around, Faith looks up."

RALPH WALDO EMERSON

January 2020

My niece sent Gary a new car calendar for Christmas. I taped it on his wall. When I pulled down the old calendar, I noticed that Gary kept track of the days by crossing each one off. In November 2019, he stopped doing this. Sorrow washed over me with the realization he no longer could. I decided to keep the new calendar up anyway.

We spent a few hours together in a nearby park, breathing in the fresh winter air. The coolness did nothing to ease his confusion. He sat in a bottomless chasm of nothingness except the knowledge that he was losing his mind. We spoke no words.

I reached over and laid my hand over his. He in turn placed his over mine. After a fair amount of silence, he said, "It is what it is."

"I'm so sorry," I empathized.

"It's not your fault," he said.

"I know. But I feel so bad. You deserve so much better."

When we returned to the facility, I noticed his prayer book on the nightstand. For as long as I could remember, Gary had kept his childhood prayer book nearby. I reached for it and noticed the binding had come loose. Instead of using the scotch tape in his room to hold it together, he had placed three band aids along the seams. I gasped with awareness. Visual reminders like this played a tug of war in my mind. *What was* and *what is*. The man I knew was fading away.

February 2020

My Self-Pity turns to Compassion

On visits with Gary, I'd chat with the resident ladies. Years of wisdom filled the bodies that weathered the sands of time. All of them were so happy to see me. I regarded them as my family. They had so much love and so many hugs to share.

I began to walk around the facility in search of Gary. There was a huge glass wall in front of the dining room. As I peeked through it, I saw people from a local Baptist church singing at the front of the room. Gospel music filled the room with joy and entertained all who were listening.

I quickly spotted Gary. He sat alone at a table, his lips moving silently to the words being sung. In that moment I didn't see dementia. I saw a man who had given so much of his life to others. I remembered the husband who never wanted to be a burden to anyone. The father who would cut off both arms for his sons. The grandfather who loved his granddaughters. The uncle who cherished time with his nieces. The man who never said no to anyone needing help. A man of God who every morning would kiss a cross that hung in our bedroom. I saw a vulnerable human being caught in the middle of a disease that was stealing the essence of his being.

A flood of compassion flowed through me like the rush of water flowing over Niagara Falls. It cleansed me of any self-pity I had been harboring on this journey. That moment—that stretch of a minute—managed to melt the ice of self-centeredness that encased me. I only felt the warmth of love for another human being.

In addition to the ice melting off my soul, the soil that embedded my feet so deep with anger, resentment, and bitterness began to loosen. It turned soft with kindness and compassion. The values that were so deeply rooted in him added to the ones embedded in me. I knew at that defining moment that no matter the difficulty of walking this journey, I would find a way to the other side of it.

From the onset of this illness Gary had asked for nothing. He was grateful and appreciative of every act of kindness extended to him. He did not utter one complaint. It was time to lessen my thoughts about the challenges of this disease and substitute them with thoughts of how he might handle it if it were me. I knew then that the Lord had chosen me for this journey, and I would honor his wishes and do whatever I could to ease Gary's suffering.

I walked into the room and took a seat next to him.

"Hi there," I said.

"Hi," he said smiling. "I'm just listening to the songs. I'm glad you came."

"Yeah, me too," I replied.

I reached over and held his hand.

March 13, 2020

I was sitting in the movie theater with a friend when my cell phone started vibrating. I ignored it. Several minutes later it repeated itself. Reluctantly, I reached for my purse. Gary was calling. Immediately I thought, *it can wait.* Gary now called dozens of times a day. Often, he didn't even know who he was calling. "Who is this?" he'd ask. But alarm bells went off in my mind when he rang a third time.

I entered the lobby to phone him. I could scarcely believe what I was hearing as he struggled to articulate what was wrong.

"They won't let me leave here!" he said frantically.

"What do you mean?" I asked.

"They said I can't leave!"

"Hang on," I said. "Calm down. Let me call the main desk and find out what's going on."

I called the assisted living facility and connected with the administrator.

"What's going on?" I asked. "Gary just called and he's very upset."

"We're so sorry, Rose, but the governor issued an order that all facilities are going on lockdown due to the Covid virus."

"Lockdown?"

"Yes, until further notice. He can't go out, and you can't come in."

"What? That can't happen. You know I'm there all the time. Gary needs to see me. He depends on me to take him on outings. He won't understand this!"

"Hopefully by the end of the month we can open the facility to the public."

"The end of the month! That's like three weeks away! I can't go a month without seeing Gary!"

"It's the governor's orders. If you want," she said, "you can see him through his window."

"Through his window?"

I could scarcely believe what I had just heard. *Three weeks! Through his window?*

I stayed rooted in the lobby. I tried to process what I had just heard. I thought of Gary's decline. *What will this mean to him?* I picked him up twice a week for outings, and on Sunday he attended church. When I visited, I checked his supplies, filled the automatic dog feeder, prepared the dogs treats, straightened up his room, and checked his clothes to make sure he didn't need anything. I had recently purchased new curtains, a bedspread, and décor that I was going to surprise him with for Easter. *Surely by Easter I'll be let in his room. If not, who would do these things?* I tried to remain calm, but the news increased my fear and anxiety. My heart bled for Gary and how the isolation would affect him.

There's absolutely no way that I can go for more than a few weeks and not pick him up. He'll be so confused! He won't be able to understand! I went into self-talk mode and reassured myself it would only be for a couple weeks. *I'll call him back when I get home. Somehow, I'll comfort him and make him understand.*

May 2020

On May 12, I received a call from the facility that Gary was not right. He was acting more confused than usual. The staff felt he was entering another stage of dementia. I had noticed when I spoke to him that morning that he could barely form a sentence. *Perhaps the isolation is starting to affect him.*

When the staff entered his room at midday, they found it askew. Gary was soaked in urine. He was tired and yawning. His vitals were normal. The care manager reached out to his primary doctor, who requested a urinalysis. She felt that Gary might have a UTI (urinary tract infection).

By late afternoon I was informed they had collected a specimen and called the laboratory for pickup. I hoped that we would know something the next day. I breathed a sigh of relief. I was already dealing with the anxiety of him not being allowed out of the facility.

The following morning, I asked the care manager if they had received any results.

She replied, "I told you a specimen was collected, and a call was made for pickup, based on something that should have happened but didn't."

I replied, "What? A specimen hasn't been taken!" My patience was wearing thin and anxiety taking over after two months of the pandemic. I also felt like I had been lied to.

She assured me they would get a specimen and forward it immediately to the laboratory, but it would take seventy-two hours to get results. One issue I had with the facility was the conflicting information I received. I always felt the need to follow up.

I called his memory care specialist, who felt if it wasn't a UTI, then perhaps it was dehydration. I phoned the care manager back and told her that his memory care specialist suggested forcing fluids in case it was dehydration. The instruction was added to his care plan.

Gary continued to get more and more confused with each day. On the morning of the fifteenth, three days after symptoms were first reported, Gary phoned and left a voicemail.

"Hi, it's Gary. I want to do something today. Anything. Please give me a call."

I decided to go to the facility and do a window visit. The care manager reported that Gary had stopped eating, so staff ordered him a nutrition shake.

An aide walked him to his open window. Gary tried to speak, but the words came out as gibberish. He was pale and in his pajamas. He looked dirty. I phoned the care manager and communicated that I did not like Gary's appearance.

I put another call into his memory care specialist, who suggested a visual exam over FaceTime. It was scheduled for the sixteenth. I tried to curb my frustration that it had now been five days since symptoms had begun, and four days since the urinalysis. *Why did the laboratory still not have results?* I had been told it took seventy-two hours, and we were now at ninety-six hours. I called the care manager numerous times, but she could not provide any additional information. My biggest fear was that if he had a UTI, it would cause sepsis.

At 5:00 p.m. on the nineteenth, eight full days after the first symptoms appeared, and after numerous follow up calls and texts, a UTI was confirmed. By this time, Gary had lost a lot of weight.

I couldn't help but be concerned about dementia patients with no advocate. Even with my vigilance, it took eight full days for an antibiotic to be prescribed. *What should I have done differently?* I always felt no matter what I did, it was never enough.

On the night of the twenty-second, I phoned Gary and noticed that he had a very slow response time. I phoned a staff member and asked that he check on Gary. He phoned back and said Gary was responding okay. I felt it strange that he did not detect what I did.

I phoned again the next morning, and Gary could barely respond to my prompts. I called the care manager. "I know something is wrong!

Call the primary." *Why had the staff not noticed this?* I received a call back that Gary was being taken to the ER for a CT and MRI to rule out a stroke. *A stroke?*

The ER concluded that he had had an allergic reaction to the antibiotic. After making sure it was added to his allergy list, I tried to relax a bit. We were now on day twelve. By 8:20 p.m., Gary was back in the ER. A resident who smoked left the door open, and Gary walked out. He fell down an embankment. I was notified EMS was called. I told the staff, "Phone the ER! Pandemic or no pandemic, I'm going in!" I sped down my mountain to the ER twenty minutes away.

The ER staff took my temperature and made sure I wore a mask. I tried to calm the anger that was raising my blood pressure. I found Gary lying on an ER cot, pale, worn, and thinner. Since the pandemic he had not had a haircut or mustache trim. His face was covered with dirt. I walked up to him and smoothed his hair back. He tried to open his eyes.

"Hi," I said. "I'm right here, sweetheart. It's going to be okay. I promise I've got this."

A nurse practitioner walked in. I started to shout, "What have you done to him? I want nothing unnecessary done to him! Do you hear me! He's been through enough! No catheters! No IVs! NOTHING." I collapsed into a chair. I had not eaten right for days. I felt my breath fall away and my thoughts out of focus.

Without saying a word, the NP sat next to me. She recognized my anger for what it was. She did not personalize it as others might have. She knew it was not directed at her. She saw the worry, anxiety, exhaustion, hopelessness, frustration, and aloneness etched on my face and the shadows from lack of sleep under my eyes. She noticed my hands trembling and my tears forcing themselves out of my eyes. Her first response was empathy. She took my hands in hers. "It's okay. It's okay. I'm right here. I'm listening. I'm so sorry."

I regurgitated everything that had happened over the last twelve days and how fraught I was with worry. I explained how alone I felt on this journey. I heard from no one. Not one call that demonstrated concern or support. I was maintaining a big house! I had to quit my job that I loved. I tried to be there for my dad. I advocated the best I could for Gary, but it never seemed to be enough!

She didn't interrupt but kept her hand in mine. When I was done draining myself of every emotion and thought, she met my tear-soaked eyes.

"I get it," she said. "I took care of my ex-husband, who had cancer. None of our children helped. It was not easy. I understand."

She continued, "I didn't do anything to Gary. What I would like to do is take a liver panel to make sure there's no ammonia in his blood that could be adding to his confusion. And I want to make sure his ribs are okay. And then we'll clean him up for you. Is that okay?"

"Yes, thank you. I'm sorry." I replied.

With the kindest eyes, she said, "It's okay. There's nothing to apologize for. Have you eaten?"

"No. I went to see my dad today. I had just gotten home when I received the call. I was going to relax and have some dinner."

She said, "Wait here."

When she returned, she had a blanket that she put around my shoulders. And then she pulled out her lunch box and shared her dinner with me. "Here," she said, as she passed a half sandwich and a bottle of water to me. "It's too much for me to eat, anyway." She sat next to me as she shared her dinner.

Gary's liver panel was fine, but he had a fractured right rib. The NP explained, "It will heal naturally. We don't tape ribs anymore. Just make sure the staff gives him Tylenol and that he takes deep breaths, so pneumonia doesn't set in. Encourage staff to put pull-ups on him so that he doesn't have to get up and down to go to the bathroom. The scans showed no bleeds, and his neck is okay. His enzymes were slightly elevated, but we won't worry about them. His face will heal but will be sore for a bit."

I returned Gary to the facility around midnight. After returning home and collapsing on my bed, I thanked the Lord for sending an angel. I would discover during this journey how many angels the Lord would send.

The next day I met with the care manager to make sure that everyone would be more attentive in getting urine samples sent in the right direction and that they be on alert for future UTIs. We found out that Gary's sample was sent to the wrong lab, which caused the delay.

June 2020

At 1:48 a.m. on June 3, an angel got her wings. I met Gail through a closed, online dementia support group. The support group comprised dementia caregivers.

Gail, an in-home caregiver, was isolated from the outside world due to the demands of caring for her mother. She had previously taken care of her dad, who had Alzheimer's. When he passed, her mom was diagnosed, and she resumed her role as caregiver.

She documented her journey and often supplied videos of her mom, so we had visuals of what each stage looked like. The caregivers on support sites have stockpiles of information on behaviors, medications, and various illnesses that go with dementia, like UTIs. Most of all, they understand and support the journey. Many on the site rant and cry, but mostly they *care* for one another—any time, any day.

It was a dark day when I went online and posted a question to the support group. Gail was the first to respond. After a few posts she messaged me, and we became online friends. I regarded her as my soul sister. It didn't matter how busy or tired she was caring for her mom, she was always there listening, sharing, and offering advice, comfort, and support.

I struggled with the lack of support I received from our family and shared my hurt. Gail said, "I have a sibling, sister-in-law, and son who live close by that rarely call or visit. I understand, Rose. You'll find many in support groups who experience what you do. We are all here for each other. Feel free to jump on anytime and share your heart. I am here for you."

Her mom passed away in January of 2020. Gail was devastated but relieved that her mom was no longer suffering. In April she began experiencing severe leg and back pain. When she got no relief from pain medications, she demanded more tests from her doctors. They found a large cancerous tumor on her spine that was fast-growing and invasive. Like many caregivers, although she had been suffering symptoms for months, she had no one to sit with her mom so that she could visit the doctor.

    She was a warrior even in this battle. Despite the grim diagnosis and both radiation and chemotherapy treatments, her light shone bright. From her hospital bed, she continued to inspire, love, and be there for anyone who needed support. Where others would crumble or bask in self-pity, Gail stood strong.

    She completed the radiation treatments, but they made her bones so frail they broke when anyone attempted to move her. Both her pelvis and leg broke. Despite her optimism and courage, cancer took her life within six months of her mother's passing.

Spread your wings, my friend, and fly high.

June 20, 2020
First Outing Since Pandemic Began

The care manager walked Gary to the car. He was unsteady and shuffled his feet. His hair was unusually long. One of the CNAs had a cosmetology license and had been trimming it since the hairstylist had not been allowed in the facility, but it still looked shaggy and unkempt. Prior to his diagnosis, Gary always went to a stylist, who kept his hair groomed. For a man his age, there were no signs of baldness or thinning. His hair still had hints of black with gray streaks.

I focused on his attire. He wore a winter shirt buttoned high up his neck. When he was younger, Gary always broke out in a sweat, even on a cool day. Since dementia he was always cold. At this stage of dementia, core body temperature is affected, and patients will often be cold. He wore his jeans tightly cinched at the waist with a belt. The belt compensated for his recent weight loss.

As he worked himself into the seat, I said, "Buckle up." He looked at me with a blank stare. The care manager said, "I've got this, Gary." She secured the seatbelt and gave him a hug. "Have a nice time, and we'll be waiting for you when you get back." I loved how the staff respected and cared for Gary. An attentive and well-trained staff is a sign of a good facility administrator.

"Thanks, I can't think these days," he responded. Pulling away, I felt I was helping someone break out of prison. This was the first outing since the pandemic began. He was allowed out for a neurologist appointment and a short visit with my sister-in-law. We would follow strict guidelines.

Prior to the pandemic, before taking Gary on an outing, I'd arrive three or four times a week and visit with a group of female residents. Sometimes I would bring my loom and yarn and show them how to knit. They loved to chat about their lives prior to entering assisted living. I heard stories of travel, careers, and the beautiful homes they owned. I considered them part of my extended family and loved sharing time with them. The pandemic halted these visits, and I missed them a lot.

I tried to compensate for the missed outings, church visits, and regular activities that took place at the facility by calling Gary three times a day, doing window visits, and bringing him takeout food. No matter how many times I explained Covid and the need to stay isolated, he forgot a moment later. "Why can't I go out again?" he'd ask. It broke my heart every time I attempted to make him understand.

I returned to the moment as I began exiting the parking lot. I saw a smile spread across his face. "It's been a long time since I did this," he shared.

"Yes, it has been," I replied. "How does it feel?"

"Good. Where are we going?"

"I have to take you to your neurologist; he's just going to check you over so he can prescribe your medication."

"Okay. And then what are we doing?"

"After the doctor I'll take you to Christi's, and we'll have a porch visit."

"Do I know Christi?"

"Yes, sweetheart. She's my sister-in-law. You'll remember her when you see her." Even though Gary and I had been separated for a decade, I still called him sweetheart or babe. During our marriage we rarely used our first names with one another. I did not want to change that. People often wonder if they should speak differently to a loved one with dementia. I never did. I still told Gary he was a pain in my butt, and it always brought a smile to his face. I felt if I stopped talking to him as I normally did, he'd stop knowing me.

As we pulled into the parking lot of the neurologist, he looked at me. "Where are you taking me?"

"To your neurologist. It's going to be okay."

It had started to drizzle, and droplets appeared on the windshield. He pointed to them.

"Look, it's tinkling," he said. Gary was now substituting a lot of words.

Once in the examination room, the neurologist approached Gary and shook his hand. After exchanging pleasantries, he noted he had seen us exactly one year prior. He appeared startled by Gary's outward decline. He asked Gary the day, month, and year and asked if he knew where he was. Gary couldn't answer any of the questions.

As was customary with these visits, he had Gary extend his arm and use his finger to touch the doctor's finger. He was assessing his coordination. Gary smiled. He was pleased with his accomplishment. The doctor then asked him to walk across the room. That concluded the examination.

Pulling into Christi's driveway, Gary smiled and said, "I know this place."

"Yes, you do," I replied. "You've been here many times."

We stayed about forty minutes, until Gary began showing signs of restlessness. He rose from the porch chair half a dozen times and then returned to his seat.

"Are you ready to go home?" I asked.

Glancing at his watch, he said, "Yes. It's time to go back." Gary could no longer tell the time. Looking at his watch was a force of habit.

As we were pulling into the facility, he said, "I think I know this place, but I'm not sure where it is."

"This is where you live, babe. You're safe here."

I was happy to have had my first outing with Gary, but witnessing someone with dementia was unlike anything I ever experienced. I had watched loved ones suffer from congestive heart failure, cancer, and liver failure. Nothing prepared me for this disease. I was now Gary's compass, helping him navigate a world he no longer knew.

Flashback

Gary always chose his words carefully. When we were with friends, he would socialize and crack jokes, but he'd never enter a conversation without knowledge, offer an opinion about something he had no experience with, or engage in idle gossip. However, if he felt what he had to say was worthy, he would jump in. He had his chance when we received a late night call from our builder.

We had purchased our first home, and Gary was very pleased that it was only half complete. He had a natural talent for building and looked forward to making a few rooms different from the architect's plans for the house. The builder assured us that he was open to change—except when we called with one. Then he would hem and haw because he knew it would put him off schedule. This was one of those nights.

Gary had sketched out with accurate measurements where he wanted an island in our kitchen. The builder called to tell Gary it was impossible. It would not provide an adequate walkway. Knowing his measurements were accurate and that it could be done, Gary challenged the builder. I could tell by Gary's face that he was becoming upset, which he rarely did. Suddenly, he instructed the builder, "This conversation is over. Meet me at the house tomorrow night at 6 p.m."

"What happened?" I asked.

"He told me my plans were a piece of shit." He fumed.

The next night he and I arrived at the house early. "Why?" I questioned.

"You'll see."

He spent the next half hour gathering a pile of two by fours and began constructing an outline of where he wanted the island placed. It had a more than adequate walkway.

When the builder walked into the kitchen, he glanced at the outline. Meeting his eyes Gary said, "Now you are going to build what I asked you to the exact specifications." As he handed him another copy of the plans, he said, "And don't you EVER call my plans shit again."

It was one of the few times I saw Gary upset. We walked out, and the island was built to Gary's specifications.

June 2020

By the end of the month, I felt the loss of control from not having more eyes on Gary or being allowed in his room. I had become very protective of him. This loss of control increased my anxiety.

When I phoned Gary, he sounded more and more confused. He'd say, "I don't know what I'm supposed to do." If I instructed him to watch TV, he'd respond, "Where is the TV?"

I'd reply, "Babe, it's the big screen on your wall."

After a pause, he'd say, "I can't find it."

If I instructed him to get a drink from his mini refrigerator, he no longer knew what it was.

I'd explain, "It's that big silver metal box at the end of your room. It has a handle. Open the door; there are drinks inside. I will wait for you. Walk across your room to it, open the door, and take a drink out."

"Okay," he'd respond.

After several minutes, he'd be back on the phone. I'd question him. "Babe, did you find it? Do you have a drink?"

"I don't know where it is," he'd answer. I'd phone the care manager and let her know that he needed someone to provide daily drinks.

I monitored songs that played on the Echo Dot in his room. When I checked Alexa on my phone to see if the songs were playing, I'd notice it was disconnected. After phoning the care manager, she'd reply, "Rose, he unplugged the clock, TV, phone and Echo Dot again."

Besides playing songs, I'd program Alexa to say things like *good morning, babe. I hope you enjoyed your breakfast.* Or *it's time to take a walk around the facility to get some exercise.* I had the staff put a note by each outlet that read, **Do Not Unplug**. The notes were not helpful. Gary could no longer read.

He was sleeping more and more. I questioned myself about keeping him at the facility during the pandemic. *Would he be better off at home?* I spoke to my therapist, who had spent her career with dementia patients and their families. She felt bringing him home would not be in his best interest. She explained. "It would put additional stress on you and would cause even more confusion in Gary. Trust me," she said. "He will not benefit from the transition."

I remember one day I decided to phone Gary. We had a fifteen-minute conversation, and, after hanging up, I stood there in utter disbelief. He sounded like Gary pre-dementia. I was happy but alarmed enough to call my therapist. I confided in her, "I don't think Gary has dementia! I've made an awful mistake. I just talked to him, and he sounded perfectly normal!" I didn't know whether to cry with joy or cry because such an awful mistake was made. She was very patient with me. "Rose, Gary has dementia. If Gary did not have dementia, he would contact his attorney, pack his bags, and call one of his friends to pick him up. Can you imagine him doing that?" Sadly, I could not.

Dementia was progressing. That coupled with the pandemic was making this journey even more difficult. I wanted to control the outcome of this disease, but of course I could not. Instead, my desire to protect Gary from the symptoms of this disease increased.

UNDERSTAND …

There is no understanding dementia.

There is no understanding people's reaction to it.

There is no understanding your reaction to it.

It's unpredictable—and varied.

Walk the journey knowing you will never understand it—and you will be okay.

You'll save yourself a lot of time questioning it.

Analyzing it.

Why did this happen?

Is this symptom normal for dementia?

How long will this stage last?

Because everyone is different.

Accept the disease and Move Forward.

June 28, 2020

First porch visit at the facility

I received a call that I could have a porch visit with Gary. I bought a couple bags of hard candy and two picture books for Gary before I picked up my 94-year-old dad to join us. I knew that would make Gary happy, as they were best buddies.

When we arrived at the facility, the outdoor porch was divided into two sections. A chair on one side was chosen for Gary, with a piece of tape showing six feet from the two facing chairs. We were instructed to leave our masks on. Our temperatures were taken and recorded. We then signed a waiver form.

It was a beautiful June day, with a breeze blowing across the porch. A staff member sat nearby to ensure that all protocols and policies were adhered to. Gary was ushered out and instructed where to sit. I was happy to see he was showered and shaved.

"Hi, babe, how ya doing?"

"Still alive and walking," he said.

"I got a milkshake for you. It's chocolate."

He reached for it and positioned the straw against the mask. I motioned for him to pull the mask down so that he could drink. He did so but tried to drink through the paper that I left on the straw.

"No, babe, pull the paper off." He was not able to process the instruction, so nearby staff helped him.

I then carried the conversation, telling him about yard work I had done, handyman repairs, and curtain panels I had hung on the porch. Gary would occasionally interject a couple words, but he had difficulty articulating complete and meaningful sentences. Dad offered a joke now and then, and Gary would laugh. Even through the clouds of dementia, he had not lost his sense of humor or his desire to make a witty or sarcastic remark. They were the few lights left in him.

We were allowed thirty minutes, but staff sitting outside let us linger longer. They understood how hard the lockdown was on residents and family and were kind and compassionate.

As dad and I headed back home, he said, "He looks good." I barely smiled. *Good?* I thought. *As compared to what?*

Three hours later I called Gary.

"What are you doing?" I asked.

He said, "I was just getting ready to go to church."

All churches were closed, it was a weekday, and Gary hadn't attended mass since the pandemic started.

"No, babe, churches are closed because of the virus."

"The virus? What's a virus?"

July 2020

The administrator at his facility was kind enough to make posters showing Gary where things were in his room. We both felt it might help him. But he tore them off the wall. He no longer knew his dog's name. He referred to Chase now as *dog*. His calls to me were more frequent, extending into the middle of the night. Gary's words were whispered and scrambled, and I had no clue what he was trying to communicate. On one call, he said his toilet was not working. I phoned an aide and asked her to check. She called me back. "The toilet is fine. He was trying to communicate that his belt buckle was broken."

I encouraged the aides to pull up his window blinds, so that Gary could distinguish between night and day. But Gary would lower them, frightened someone would see into his room. If it rained, he was afraid the rain would come through the closed window. Or he was afraid the cold could get in even though it was summer.

Most nights I cried myself to sleep. I grieved for the loss of my best friend. I would have written a check for any amount for a five-minute conversation with him. I'd lie in bed and whisper to the empty air, *I miss you so much, babe.*

Staff reported that mornings were getting more difficult for Gary. He struggled to walk the dog or make his bed. Assistance with showering, shaving, and brushing his teeth had started six months prior. After getting dressed and taking his dog out into the courtyard, he'd return to his room. It was not unusual for me to call at 10 a.m. and find he was back in bed. He simply did not know what to do with himself. I encouraged him to walk the hallways for exercise, and he'd agree to do that and thank me for the suggestion.

Because of the pandemic, residents could not congregate in groups. Activities such as bingo were limited to the hallways, with residents sitting outside their rooms. Prior to the pandemic Gary had only participated in a few activities. He felt more comfortable in his room with his dog. Staff would encourage him to join in, but they could not force him. I requested that a social worker from the psych team and one from palliative care visit Gary. But the visits were only a couple times a month.

Dining was an activity that Gary enjoyed, and it broke his day into three parts. Meals were served at 7:30 a.m., 12:30 p.m., and 5:30 p.m. However, residents were now forced to eat in their rooms, which increased Gary's isolation. He forgot he was supposed to stay in his room and walked down to the dining room at mealtimes. Because no one else was there, the facility allowed him to stay.

Many times, when I phoned Gary, he'd be upset that Chase had broken out of his harness. Gary could no longer put it on Chase correctly, so I instructed staff to leave the harness on Chase. While walking Chase, if something caught Gary's attention, he would drop the leash. Staff would then need to chase after the dog. The disruption upset Gary. He was petrified they would take his dog away. One day staff reported that when Chase broke loose Gary said, "He hurt my feelings." On more than one occasion, in trying to discipline the dog, Gary would swipe at him. Staff interceded and cautioned Gary not to hit the dog.

I decided one day to surprise Gary with a visit from the doorway out front. My conversations with Gary were one-sided. "You look good. I picked up some roast beef sandwiches for you. I see you got a shower today; your hair looks nice and clean. Are you enjoying your day? It's so nice out."

When I asked, "Are you okay?" He'd answer, "I'm still walking and talking." His mouth and nose were hidden by a mask, but I saw his eyes smile. He tried to share a witty or sarcastic comment, but dementia had robbed his ability to do so. He'd begin and then not be able to finish. I'd note the frustration on his face.

As I headed home, I received a call from Gary.

"Hi, babe. What's up?"

"Are you supposed to be coming today?"

Not visiting a person with dementia because they will forget the visit a short while later is not a reason to stay away. While you are with them, they feel loved. It's really all they have left. Their heart remembers a scent, a touch, a hug, a smile, a phrase you used to say, a name you used to call them, and they enjoy listening to memories of who they were.

July 14, 2020

I received permission to take Gary to an appointment with his memory care specialist. I was so happy to see Gary, but I couldn't help but notice how frail he looked.

At the specialist's office, I made small talk with Gary. Then an assistant ushered Gary into a room for his mental status exam. After half an hour, she came to get me. "Gary is very anxious and wants to go home," she said. I walked into the exam room, and he got up to leave.

"Hang on a second, babe, we're just going to talk to the doctor."

"I want to leave," he said as he walked down the hall.

I caught up and began coaxing him. "I promise, we'll only be a few more minutes. Please come back with me. When we leave here, I'll treat you to a milkshake."

He complied with my request but was clearly anxious.

The doctor recorded his weight at 180 pounds and noted his vitals were good. She reported that his speech was low volume with word-finding difficulty. Insight into his cognitive deficits was fair. His eyes were closed for much of the visit. He had difficulty rising from a seated position, and his gait was slightly stooped and slow but steady, with low foot clearance and reduced arm swing. Memory was impaired, mood was flat with muted affect, and his thoughts were goal directed.

She reported that Gary told her he was "losing his memory, he's angry at his loss, and said that his dog is his life." He repeatedly told her it was time to go home and check on his dog. When asked if he felt he was well cared for, he replied, "Yes."

My eyes filled as I read through the rest of the test results. Gary was losing ground. My days were always filled with hope that the disease would stop. I forced the frown from my face so Gary would not notice. I made the decision that this would be the final visit. I explained to the specialist, "Gary gets upset doing these examinations. Why continue? It's obvious that Gary is declining. No medication will help him return to his former self." The memory specialist agreed with me. I tried to accept the fact that this was what dementia did, but grief saturated my heart. Grief that I was losing Gary, and that Gary was losing himself.

"Come on, babe. Let's get a milkshake and sit at the lake for a while. We're done here."

He walked to the car with head downcast. *What was he thinking?*

August 9, 2020

I phoned the facility's corporate office and told them Gary's health was declining due to isolation. "If you do not allow me to take him out, he will die. Neither one of us wants that," I pleaded. Corporate allowed me compassionate care. I was able to take him outside the facility using cautionary measures such as wearing a mask and keeping him a safe distance from others. I could not enter the facility, but staff could meet me outside.

I was very happy that I could resume our outings. I notified the staff I'd be picking up Gary but cautioned them not to tell him. He would become anxious and call me a dozen times before I arrived.

A staff member was waiting outside with Chase, and another guided Gary to the car. I was glad he was dressed in a short sleeve t-shirt; it was over 90 degrees. I got used to the sweat dripping off me as Gary would be cold if I ran the air conditioner.

As we drove away, he asked, "Where are you taking me?"

"We're just going over to Christi's. Punky and Chase can run in the yard."

"Who's Chase?" He asked.

"Our dog. He's in the car." I replied.

He glanced at the back seat. "Where is he?" he asked frantically.

"Babe, he's in the back seat. He's right behind you. You can't see him."

He looked relieved. "Where are you taking me again?"

"Over to Christi's." I willed myself to be patient with the repetitiveness.

"I'm getting weaker," he said sorrowfully.

"Weaker physically? Or weaker mentally?"

"I can't think anymore."

"I'm so sorry. I can't imagine how frustrating it must be."

"Soon you won't have to worry about me anymore. Where are you taking me again?"

Despite the repetitiveness and memory loss, I still enjoyed taking Gary out and spending special times with him. I was happy to be able to add some joy to his life.

September 2020

On Labor Day, I received a second contract on my mountain home. It was twenty years to the day since we had moved into our dream home. My fourteen-year journey of trying to sell this property on and off was coming to an end. This contract, unlike before, appeared solid.

With a contract came the ordeal of another inspection. This inspector ran so much water it ran my well dry. My HVAC system needed a repair, but I was grateful when I learned it was minor. I had 30 days to complete a ton of paperwork, pack up the house, sell furniture, schedule movers, and most importantly find a new home during a pandemic.

Each room in that house whispered happy memories with Gary. It was emotionally exhausting walking through each room and packing. I also had to go through all of Gary's belongings, and he wasn't even dead. I placed his memorabilia in a box that I would later go through and share with both his sons.

The pandemic depleted the market in western North Carolina. It appeared everyone wanted to move to the mountains where there were fewer people. I was convinced that the city of Asheville, one and a half hours from Gary, was where I wanted to be. Even though it would increase travel time for visits, Asheville was more citified. I was ready to be closer to shops and to people regardless of the pandemic.

I made a list of what I wanted in my home. I wanted it to be in a loving and supportive neighborhood. It had to be new, one story, low maintenance, fenced yard, two bedrooms, two baths, an office, and a screened-in porch. My realtor friend chuckled. "You do know, Rose, this is virtually impossible in today's market." However, she found me a home that met all the criteria within a couple of weeks. I know the Lord played a part in this.

In October, I moved and everything that could have gone wrong during a pandemic did. All the furniture I ordered was backordered and then canceled. Other things I ordered arrived broken, the wrong color, or not as described. Even though the house was new, there was a list of minor tasks that needed to be completed by the builder. But when I settled in, I was able to breathe a sigh of relief. I knew I was heading in the right direction.

As exhausted as I was, the next day I drove an hour and a half to share the news with Gary that I was in a new home. He appeared to understand, smiled, and said, "Good."

We took a short walk and sat on a bench. He tired so quickly. My heart was burdened with the knowledge that I was moving forward, and he was moving backward. *How is this fair, Lord?* Talking through his mask, he said, "I'm not getting better."

"Babe..."

"No, it's okay, I know. I know I'm not getting better. I can tell."

My tears, my constant companion, started to flow. I forced myself to concentrate on the river in front of me. I envisioned it carrying the memories of our life together further and further from the shore. I wanted to build a dam to stop it midstream. *Just stop!* I heard my heart shout. I looked over at Gary.

"Don't cry," he said.

"I'm so sorry. I want to fix this. If I had a magic wand, I'd wave it over you and make it okay. I would, babe. I just don't know what else to do."

"I know," he said.

On this journey, I felt more and more despair with each visit. It's hard to feel so helpless. It would have been so much easier if I had had someone to share visits with. I was anguished all the time about what I could do to help him. I felt guilty if I had a good day. *Why him, why not me?* As much as I told myself, *it's not your fault,* I felt uncomfortable that I was well, and he was not. That I could enjoy my life and he could not. *Survivor's guilt.*

December 2020

The assisted living facility allowed me into Gary's room for the first time since the pandemic began. I went through his armoire and discarded unwanted clothes and hung new drapes, a bedspread, and bathroom décor. I decorated his room for the holiday. I noticed his room seemed less clean, but I expected it as so many staff left during the pandemic.

I pounded my steering wheel from grief on the way home. Gary was even more confused, and it was getting harder for him to contain his emotions. "I just can't think anymore! I can't do anything! I just want to kill myself." I thought of the many caregivers online who after witnessing this journey state, "I'll kill myself if I'm ever diagnosed."

Gary no longer knew what he was supposed to be doing. He felt totally lost in the world he lived in. He knew one day he'd not even know who he was. He shared, "one day I won't even recognize myself in the mirror." The compass that directs the life of a human being is nonexistent or distorted with dementia. Nothing in the world makes sense.

I tried to support and encourage him, but even that was getting more difficult. I'm a realist. I wasn't going to say, "It's going to get better." Or "we'll find someone who can make you better." I knew that was not going to happen. I couldn't lie to him. And I certainly was not going to make light of his situation. Instead, I made sure he knew that, no matter what, I'd always be at his side. I'd tell him, "Even if you don't know I am here, I will be. I promise. I know it's hard, but just do the best you can. And I'll help you as much as I can." He appeared comforted when I said that. I was the only compass he had.

It had been two and a half years since Gary was diagnosed. The clock was ticking. Would anyone phone to say they'd like to visit for the holidays? How many years did he have left? Did it matter only to me?

My mind returned to happier times. In one memory, Christmas was a couple days away, and our ten-year-old son decided there was no Santa Claus. Gary and I wanted to keep the fantasy alive for him, as he had lost so many holidays during his years in foster care. Steve said, "Okay, Mom, if there's a Santa Claus, he will put a big red bow on the top of Dad's new boat."

On Christmas Eve, Gary and I stood outside in the dark next to the boat sitting on a trailer. There was snow and ice on the ground, and we both knew Gary would need a ladder to secure a bow to the top. I held the ladder as Gary climbed to the top and secured the bow. He wasn't satisfied.

He took a sled from the garage and carried it and the ladder to the back of the house. Climbing that ladder with the sled, he positioned it on the flat roofline outside Steve's window. Back and forth he pushed that sled to make Santa tracks in the snow.

The next morning, Steve was surprised but skeptical. "I guess maybe he does exist." The fantasy was kept alive for another year.

Christmas was always a festive day. I'd spend weeks pouring through cookbooks looking for a different theme for dinner. The house would be decorated and lit up. After the gifts were opened, Gary would do all the chopping and cutting for dinner. I was the cook, but he never hesitated to help me prepare. The table would be set with my Gorham Secret Garden China, gold-plated flatware, and silver and gold bow napkin rings. Colorful streamers would hang from the chandelier. A menu would be displayed on the table letting the family know what to expect. One year the theme was Italian, another year Amish. Every year was different. After Christmas, we would visit Gary's son and his family.

Since returning to our mountain home in 2014, the holiday was much lower key. Gary and I would meet the family at Dad's church. I prepared food to bring to Dad's. I'd arrive early to set up a small Christmas tree on the dining room table and make things as festive as possible. I'd bring gifts for everyone. Although it wasn't the same as the years we shared when Steve was a child, I adapted to holidays with my brothers and dad.

Christmas 2020 came and went. No visits or calls from our sons or their families. I sat in my new home alone on a lounge chair in the back room. It snowed that day, so I opted to bring dinner to Gary and Dad after the holiday. A family member texted that it was awful that I would not be seeing my dad on Christmas day. *He'll be so lonely!* I wondered, *What about Gary? He's always alone. What about me? I'm always alone on this journey.* It perplexed me how little thought was given to the two people experiencing so much aloneness and suffering.

Another year would be starting, and I did my best to put faith in the Lord that he would get Gary and me through it. I was learning quickly that dementia didn't wait for anyone. For those waiting for the perfect time to visit, I knew it had already passed.

Gary's symptoms – end of 2020
Moderate dementia

- He can no longer find the words he needs.
- His physical challenges are adding to his confusion.
- Blank stares and half masked eyes are more common.
- Sleep, sleep, more sleep.
- Staff reports he's crying more.
- His memory is less than a ten-minute retention.
- He calls throughout the day and night. His speech is gibberish.
- He shuffles his feet.
- He can no longer secure his seatbelt.
- He finds it helpful for me to tell him what to do.
- He can no longer harness the dog.
- He lets everyone know, "All I do is walk these halls all day."
- He engages less and less.
- Common sentences: "I can't think!" "What's my name?"
- He wants to find his people (his heart wants to feel the love from the people he can no longer identify with).
- He lets me and others know he no longer wants to live.

- He whispers.
- He knows he's not going to make it.
- He is fearful of almost everything.
- He is always cold.
- He unplugs everything in his room.
- He cannot find the mini refrigerator or TV (he no longer knows what they are called).
- He no longer watches TV.
- He does not recognize the building he lives in.
- He shaved off the mustache he had worn for fifty years (the hair on his face bothered him.).
- He can scrawl out his name, but he does not know it.
- He knows his social security number, but he has no idea what social security is.

His heart knows me, and he always expresses gratitude.

Anticipatory Grief

As if Gary's dementia, the financial strain of the disease, undeserved guilt, and desertion of family weren't enough, anticipatory grief was settling into my bones. Gary was given five years when he was diagnosed. If that were accurate, he had two years left. The grief and the fear of what lay ahead kept me awake at night. Ahead of the looming death, the anticipation of Gary's demise consumed me.

Even though I was processing the disconnect from family and the weariness of watching a loved one drift away, I was still committed to my promise to stay by Gary's side. I felt myself encapsulated in never ending grief. I'd make plans to get away for a day, and the facility would call with another crisis. I'd be at a movie, and a call would come in. Caregivers on support groups always share, "I had to cancel my plans yet again."

If given the opportunity, *would I have passed the baton?* I certainly mentioned it a few times to family when exhaustion set in. "Take the reins anytime," I'd encourage. However, in a race you are confident that the next runner will grab hold of that baton and without any instruction take it and run to the finish line. I had no one in my life who could do that. How do you provide years of instruction and expect someone to pick up midstream? Because I had already invested so much in care, I could not walk away. The anxiety of Gary not getting the care I wanted for him and the guilt of breaking my promise would haunt me.

I started experiencing symptoms of anticipatory grief, anger with the disease, and anxiety. My anger would be triggered by any number of different emotions caused by the disease. Stress, impatience, tiredness, loneliness, frustration, irritation, and unfairness. I'd explode like a firecracker when it's met with a match. Where once I'd been patient in traffic, I'd now curse and beat my steering wheel. If I was disappointed because I needed to cancel more plans, I'd exhaust myself ranting or raving. I hung up on people who were not attentive to my needs, ripped up to-do lists into tiny little shreds, and could not focus long enough to read a page in a book. Where once I would have apologized for poor behavior, I rarely cared anymore what people thought. If they *knew* what was going on, they'd understand. And if they didn't care enough to *know*, I was ready to write them off. I thought, you're either part of my life during the bad, or you won't be part of my life during the good.

Anxiety and its faithful companion *fear* followed me every day. Calls from the facility, another medical bill, or a statement on when benefits would run out triggered these feelings. If it were a really bad day, I'd take refuge under a blanket wishing I could just hide from it all. The ringtone on my phone made me break out in a cold sweat. So, I would hide my phone and then get anxious because I forgot where it was hidden. I'd circle a hospital parking lot for a half hour talking myself through the door to be there for Gary. Anxiety gripped me so hard and so fast in the dark of night I'd will myself to breathe—*just breathe, Rose, just breathe.* And when I was able, and I searched for sleep, the only thing I found was tears. Tears for Gary—and tears for myself.

I grieved every time I saw the decline that was putting Gary one step closer to his grave. It was frequent and gut wrenching. Anticipating how he would die was a living nightmare. Would he have a death rattle? Would he be bedbound and need to be hoisted out of bed like a quadriplegic? Would his seizures become uncontrollable? Would he lose the capacity to swallow and choke on his own saliva? Would he go blind? Would he get bed sores? Would he break a bone and not be able to endure surgery? These were all possibilities with late-stage dementia. I felt I was in quicksand being dragged to the bottom of a bottomless pit. I asked the Lord to take Gary quickly and easily. And then I felt guilty for having asked.

If I began sharing with family members my feelings of anger, exhaustion, grief, or abandonment, they would personalize my anger and feel it was directed at them or their loved one. They would project whatever they were feeling in defense of themselves or others. I expected empathy, but they felt the need to justify their positions. I learned early on that there are very few people who have good listening ears. Perhaps guilt and lack of participation in the journey put some in a defensive rather than empathetic mode. And then there were those who acted very blasé about my suffering. *Well, that's what dementia is like.* Really? And how would you know that? I thought.

One way to get through grief is to express it. I knew as a clinical social worker that I needed to express my pain to ward off depression. Being a private person, I did not always feel secure sharing my personal life. I was usually the person people came to. I wasn't comfortable with the role reversal. Sharing my grief would expose a vulnerable part of myself. I present myself as a person of strength. I didn't want to imply to others that I was a weakling.

Therapy helped me process my pain. I had a wonderful therapist who had spent most of her life as a memory care specialist. But journeying through dementia and dealing with daily challenges were time consuming and difficult. Regurgitating it all in a therapy session was exhausting.

So, I found myself talking to myself a lot. I was a therapist, after all, so I found myself thinking like one. I worked through different emotions as they surfaced. I forced myself to think positively and asked the Lord to help Gary in his suffering. I quelled my anxiety about the future, which I had no control over. I'd ask myself, *what's the worst that could happen?* and then put myself in problem solving mode. I took long walks and watched what I ate. I increased my meditation in the morning. And I realized that the longer I was on this journey, the more strength I gained. If Gary wasn't playing the role of victim, neither would I.

Invisible patients
The struggle for dementia sensitivity in medical care

"If you believe very strongly in something,
stand up and fight for it."

ROY T. BENNETT
The Light in the Heart

UTIs

Urinary tract infections (UTIs) are very common with dementia. Because dementia makes the brain vulnerable, it puts a person's physical health at higher risk. Also, poor hygiene, age, diminished neurological function, and/or living in a facility increase the chance of infections.

UTIs can quickly produce symptoms such as aggression, delirium, and confusion. Often there are no physical signs, such as abnormal urine, output frequency, odor, or pain. Infections can affect appetite, increase the risk of falls, and produce a decline in function. The symptoms worsen if not treated quickly. If they are undertreated, bacteria will enter the lower urinary tract, causing sepsis.

During Gary's eight months of infections (February–September 2021) he had multiple ER visits and was admitted to four different hospitals. In addition, he had outpatient tests, procedures, and surgeries.

If dementia patients are left to fend for themselves, they might be subjected to unnecessary tests, neglect, and possibly abuse. It is extremely important for the caregiver and/or POA to file reports to the hospital's CEO if they feel their loved one has been mistreated. It will protect the next patient.

Dementia demands advocates in medical environments. I witnessed the lack of dementia knowledge and sensitivity from medical professionals. A properly trained professional demonstrates verbal and nonverbal communication competency, responds to a patient assertively, not aggressively, and practices acceptable touching. They also learn techniques for redirecting patients, handling confusion, and deescalating aggressive patients with nonpharmacologic approaches.

Specialized dementia training results in patients experiencing better communication with providers and positive outcomes on psychological and behavioral systems. Psychological systems involve emotions, cognitive functions, and mental processes. Behavioral symptoms in dementia patients will appear as anxiety, agitation, and aggression. Understanding these systems empowers a provider to address them

A journey of love

effectively by providing compassionate care, skills to manage difficult symptoms, thereby enhancing a patient's well-being. Cost, the time necessary to train, or urgency to fill positions are never valid reasons to place dementia patients in the hands of untrained medical professionals.

At the time Gary was diagnosed with dementia, I did not realize that dementia disturbs bodily functions. Gary always enjoyed excellent physical health, so I did not give this aspect of his health a second thought. When his body began to malfunction and required hospitalization, I was appalled to see that he was treated as if he were invisible.

Advocating for patients during hospitalizations was not new to me, because in the past I had been present for my parents, but those experiences paled in comparison to Gary's journey. My parents were able to speak, ask questions, voice concerns, and object to procedures when I was not present. They had normal, functioning brains. Patients with dementia do not have these benefits.

I was always puzzled when family questioned why it was necessary for me to stay with a grown man during an ER visit or hospitalization. Even when I explained that Gary had the mental capacity of a four-year old, they needed further explanation and offered no empathy for the exhaustion I felt providing coverage alone. Nor did anyone volunteer to help.

At the time I was naïve to facility policies and protocols that would dictate whether Gary could continue to reside in what he considered his home. I had no learning curve; I needed to jump in and learn quickly. I was blessed with a voice that demanded attention.

February 2021

At 7:30 a.m., Gary was transported to the ER from his assisted living facility because he was not responding well to questions. The facility suspected a UTI and had performed a urinalysis a couple days before. The facility was waiting for the results, which took 72 hours.

En route to the hospital, I notified EMS that Gary's urine was sitting in the hospital lab and to make sure the attending physician received the information. I did not want them to insert a catheter in Gary unnecessarily. It's a very traumatic procedure for someone with dementia, especially if a loved one is not present. He could be aggressive because of fear and the inability to process what they were doing.

Upon entering Gary's ER cubicle, I noticed a pool of blood on the floor. Immediately I tensed. Gary looked pale as he rested on the ER cot.

A nurse entered the cubicle. "Gary did not like the straight catheter we inserted for a urine sample."

"What? I notified EMS that Gary's urine is in the laboratory. I want to see the on-call doctor immediately!" Feeling like a volcano ready to erupt, I attempted to control my anger.

Several minutes later, the doctor walked in with his head downcast.

"Excuse me. Why would you insert a catheter into my husband with moderate dementia when I phoned the EMS that a urine sample was in your lab?"

"I didn't get that information," he said.

Standing in front of him, I dialed EMS.

After asking the necessary questions, EMS provided the answer I wanted to hear.

"I'll call the ER myself and straighten this out. We take pride in relaying information that is given to us. I told them when I brought your husband in that a urine sample was in their lab."

I informed the doctor I would be filing a report with the CEO. *During the investigation the doctor relayed he took another sample because he wanted to make sure it was clean. Urine samples are taken routinely at assisted living facilities.*

Incompetency/Insensitivity during discharge

After a night of IV antibiotics, Gary was set for discharge the next morning. A CNA (certified nursing assistant) entered his room. I asked her for help in getting Gary washed and dressed. Without a word to Gary, she lowered his bed to a flat position and pulled the urine pad out from under him. She grabbed the washcloth I had prepared in the sink and wiped him off, offering no words of comfort or direction. Her behavior mimicked wiping down a doll instead of a seventy-eight-year-old man.

"He's too wiggly," she said abruptly. "I'm going to get someone to help me dress him."

"His name is Gary," I said. I wanted to tell her how to speak to a dementia patient, but I refrained. *Let's see how she behaves when someone is present.*

She returned with her assistant and together they were able to dress him.

I then asked her, "Can you help him brush his teeth?"

"You can take him to the sink and do it." she said. I took Gary to the sink and finished her job.

When she returned to the room, she said to her aide, "You'll have to help me get this one in the car." I was appalled by her language and the way she referred to my husband.

"Excuse me," I interrupted. "I told you his name was Gary." She ignored me.

I made a full report by email to the CEO. I was told other complaints were lodged against this CNA. The head nurse asked if I wanted to file an incident report. "Absolutely," I responded. I wanted to make sure future patients were protected.

During another hospitalization, I reported this CNA again. I walked into the room to find Gary throwing up mouthwash that he drank. He was not instructed properly and monitored. He thought it was water. I also found my husband naked and shivering on a shower bench while this CNA shaved him.

"Can you please cover my husband with something?" I asked. "He is cold."

My request was ignored.

Why a caregiver must be present

Within a few days of discharge Gary was readmitted to the hospital. I phoned his son and told him I needed help pulling ten-hour shifts. Ralph agreed to come for a few days. Rarely does a hospital have someone to assist patients with toileting, feeding, etc. Depending on the stage of dementia, a patient is not able to articulate that they need help. They do not know or remember how to use a call button. One must not assume that medical staff members have knowledge of dementia or dementia sensitivity training. Unfamiliar environments will increase confusion, agitation, and possibly aggression in dementia patients, so it is imperative that a familiar face be present during the day and possibly the night.

Ralph arrived in time to hear the news that his dad's diminished neurological function was not allowing him to empty his bladder completely. The urine that remained was causing his UTIs. A suprapubic catheter was suggested because a confused dementia patient is prone to pull out a foley (a tube inserted into the urethra), which could cause serious damage. A suprapubic catheter is a hollow tube inserted into the bladder through a cut in the stomach. It is performed under a local anesthetic.

Gary had a difficult time post-surgery understanding the pain and his inability to urinate normally. He needed gentle, consistent reminders of what had happened to his body every half hour to alleviate his fear, prevent him from pulling the catheter, and help with his confusion. Because of the IV in his right hand, he needed assistance with feeding. He was set for discharge within a few days, so I quickly found and hired two sitters at $20 an hour to be with him 24/7 for 4 days. Assisted living does not provide the one-on-one supervision that Gary needed while he recuperated.

Witnessing dementia insensitivity

Within two days of discharge, the facility doctors noticed Gary's suprapubic was defective and phoned EMS. When I entered the ER, the on-call urologist had approached Gary with the news that he needed a foley catheter. Her voice was far from soothing and calming.

As his POA, I instructed, "My husband does not know what a foley is. He has moderate dementia."

Ignoring me, she began instructing Gary to take a deep breath.

I met her eyes. "Can you explain to him what you are doing or provide a mild sedative?"

"I do not have time for that! I have other patients."

Holding Gary's hands, I looked into his eyes, "Okay, sweetheart, we can do this." I demonstrated by taking a deep breath. She began inserting the catheter, allowing him no time to relax or process. He began to thrash and scream. She instructed a large male nurse to hold him down. A caregiver never forgets the screams or the panic in a loved one's eyes.

"You are traumatizing him! Gary has the mental capacity of a four-year-old," I shouted.

Ignoring me, she finished the insertion. It appeared more painful than most and drew blood.

"Are you kidding me? Is that the best you could do? Have you no dementia sensitivity?"

She began, "If he took a deep breath, it wouldn't have hurt as much."

I attempted to process the lack of dementia sensitivity for her patient. When I learned that he'd be returning to the facility with a large urine bag and not one that was attached to his leg, I phoned Gary's primary doctor at the facility. She wanted him admitted for monitoring; the urologist disagreed. "We don't have sitters at the hospital, and he'll do better if returned to familiar surroundings." It surprised me that doctors in hospitals knew little about facility care, and facility doctors knew little about hospital care.

Lack of hospital sitters

The second suprapubic procedure was scheduled two days later. Gary and I waited all day to be taken into outpatient surgery. They finally took him in at 5:30 p.m. For an average patient, the wait is exhausting. But for a dementia patient it's agony. He was not allowed food or drink the entire day, he needed to stay in place and was not allowed to walk around. He was very frightened of the new surroundings. I did my best to calm his nerves and entertain him for nine and a half hours.

After the procedure, he was bleeding so badly they had to admit him. He now had both a suprapubic and a foley catheter. When I returned the next morning, I found him heavily sedated. I was told by a nurse he was given Haloperidol. It is an antipsychotic drug FDA approved for schizophrenia and bipolar disorder. It heavily sedates a patient and stays in their system for days. It is standard protocol for dementia patients to keep them in place because hospitals lack sitters.

It took hours until the drug wore off enough that I could assist him in getting dressed. No instructions were left by the urologist on when the foley could be removed and a half dozen of my calls went unanswered. The nurses' attempts to reach the urologist were also unsuccessful. Gary and I left the hospital with no pain medication or instructions.

Facility care

Most assisted living facilities would not have allowed Gary back because of this new medical need. But the administrator and the staff where he resided all loved Gary and assumed his situation was temporary. However, I needed to hire sitters again to provide one-on-one supervision while he recuperated.

Doctors Making House Calls (a group practice) assigned to the facility was concerned enough about his scrotum to do a FaceTime video. An order was put in for Tramadol for pain. Palliative care agreed to come to the facility to remove the foley. The administrator at the facility was able to make a referral to home health. *If I had Gary at home, I would not have been able to get help on board so quickly.*

Despite additional calls to the urologist who performed the surgery I did not receive a call back until two days after his discharge. I expressed my disappointment at her lack of follow-up.

"I left you a voice message!" she replied rudely.

"No, you did not. It is nowhere on my phone." I said.

"Then your phone is broken," she informed me.

I chuckled. "You mean the one I am speaking on?"

Walking a Tightrope

I prayed daily that I would have the courage and strength to support Gary. You must wear very thick skin to advocate for a loved one with medical professionals who are at times aloof and not dementia sensitive. This journey of raw, roller coaster emotions affect a person's mental health. The constant decision-making, advocating, care managing, working with insurance companies, and financing the journey contribute to a caregiver's mental and physical exhaustion.

I found when dealing with medical professionals my voice and tone needed to be deferential. The questions I asked needed to be non-intimidating, without a hint of anger or disrespect. This was extremely difficult when emotions were raw. If I behaved or spoke any other way, they would turn and walk away. Many times, I saw little empathy or bedside manner.

I became very protective of Gary. If I saw him being mishandled or managed like a piece of meat rather than a vulnerable human being with the mentality of a child, my anger rose before it could be tamed. I questioned why my input was not taken seriously by professionals. I had known this person longer than they. So why was no one listening to me?

It's very hard to keep emotional balance while being tugged in many directions. Even more so when you cannot get information or answers that are needed to properly advocate for someone. In the wee hours of the morning, I wanted to fall into a chasm of nothingness, forget this nightmare and all the demands of it.

April 2021

Insensitivity toward patient & caregiver

Gary was scheduled for his second suprapubic catheter change. They were very painful, but Gary endured. After we left the office, I took Gary to a nice lunch, determined to provide some joy. As I was buckling him into the car for our ride back to the facility, I checked his urine bag. It was empty! What? I immediately called the urologist and raced back to the office. I was in utter disbelief. I fought to quell the anxiety of what this meant.

After examination, the urologist realized he did a false insertion. He tried to get another catheter in by using a camera, but Gary fought him. It was too painful, and Gary did not understand what was going on. The urologist had no other choice but to close off the suprapubic and insert a foley catheter. I was furious! *Two suprapubic surgeries for nothing! How could this be?*

After I told the urologist how I felt, he just shrugged his shoulders and walked off. He literally left me standing there holding a urine bag. This was a medical professional who performed a catheter insertion incorrectly. He behaved like he just used the wrong type of band aid. No apologies. No answers. No nothing. I stood in disbelief, trying to regain my composure. I would not allow Gary to see me upset after what he had just experienced. Secretly I cursed the urologist to whom I had entrusted Gary's care.

Walking through the parking lot with a urine bag in tow, anxiety gripped me. Would this cause the facility to evict Gary? This was no longer a temporary situation. I had no idea how long he would require a foley.

Dementia caregivers live with chronic anxiety accompanied by fear. I was already experiencing symptoms of irritability, hypervigilance, fatigue, racing thoughts, and feelings of impending doom. I was becoming as worried about my own health as I was about Gary's.

May 2021

Facility Reacts

A couple weeks later, the administrator called me into her office.

"Rose, we are out of compliance because of Gary's foley. You need to transfer him to a nursing facility or hire a private nurse. He needs foley checks at least three times a week."

"Huh?"

She replied, "I'm sorry. I love Gary, but I cannot have our facility out of compliance."

"Are you kidding me?! This is Gary's home. It is not in his best interest to move him!"

"Rose, it HAS to be done."

Despite my emotional drain, I began calling nursing facilities, but there were wait lists, and most did not have locked down units for dementia patients. Transitioning Gary at this time would be very hard on him. Skilled nursing would increase his cost of care by $3,500 a month. Besides his foley, Gary had no other medical needs.

A traveling nurse would cost between $1,200 to $1,500 a month for three one-hour checks per week at his current facility. I hired my friends spouse who was an RN to provide the catheter checks at $700 a month. This would keep the facility in compliance and keep Gary at home. I felt it was the better choice.

Ladybug

It was a beautiful day when I decided to pick up Gary and treat him to lunch. We had hibachi chicken, soba noodles, and carrots. I relaxed in the moment, ignoring the odd eating habits Gary had acquired. He began each meal by mixing up all the food on his plate. If there was dessert nearby, he'd add it to the food. As he ate, I tried not to concentrate on the jumbled-up mess he had created. I was pleased that he still had a good appetite.

After lunch, I decided to take him for a drive into Smoky Mountain Park. We were blessed to see a huge elk standing alongside the road. I pulled over so that Gary could have a closer look. He got so excited.

His eyes were wide as he said, "We're riding through a forest. Isn't it a wonderful world?"

"Yes, it is, sweetheart."

With dementia everything one sees appears new. Gary now noticed the color of the sky, the height of the mountains, and the bright green of the trees. He was like a child seeing these things for the first time.

I stopped at a store selling outdoor decor. I helped Gary out of the car and held his arm. I noticed how unsteady he was becoming. We worked our way into the shop. He stopped and chose a colorful metal ladybug that could be staked into the ground. He reached for a nonexistent wallet.

"I want to buy this for you." he said.

"Thank you, sweetheart! That's so nice of you. I have your money."

"I want to do it. You have my money?"

"Yes. You have money but I keep it for you. I want it to be safe."

"Okay." He watched, perplexed, as I pulled out a debit card.

"What's that?" he asked.

"It has your money on it. It's better than carrying cash."

"Really?"

The reality of how much knowledge he was losing always made me sad.

Just enjoy the sweetness of the day, I told myself.

June 2021
Dementia Insensitivity

The UTIs and bladder spasms continued. I found another urologist for a second opinion. When we arrived at his office, I was already on edge. Gary had uncomfortable bladder spasms the whole way in.

After introductions, I got the urologist up to date.

He began, "I feel it might be a prostate and not a bladder issue. A procedure called a TURP (transurethral resection of prostate) might help Gary. I'll need to perform another cystoscopy."

I was immediately concerned. "Gary does not do well after any anesthesia."

"I'll give him a twilight medication. I'll be in and out as quickly as I can," he said encouragingly.

"I'll think about it," I replied, still concerned.

After the consultation, I had Gary's private nurse stay with him for a catheter change. If left in place too long it increases the likelihood of infection. I retreated to the waiting room as I could not witness another insertion. From the waiting room, I heard Gary's screams. I immediately began to shake as my eyes welled with tears. I got up and began to pace. I wanted to race back in, but I knew if I were going to survive this journey that I needed to protect my emotions. I heard Gary scream again. I walked up to the nurse's station.

"What is going on in there?" I demanded. "Why is my husband screaming?"

"It's okay. Please try to relax," she instructed.

"You're kidding, right?" My husband is screaming, and you want me to relax?" I paced the waiting room, walked outside, and returned, praying that it was finished. I was finally told I could go into the doctor's office. I could barely walk. My legs felt like rubber. My stomach was in a knot. Bile sat in my throat.

As I walked down the hall, Gary appeared from the other direction. He was very pale. He stared ahead like a zombie. He could barely walk unassisted. I felt I had betrayed him. I hugged him tight and had a difficult time letting go. While the memory of his screams would be etched in my mind forever, they had already left Gary's. I looked over at his private nurse.

"What the hell happened in there?"

She shrugged her shoulders nonchalantly. *Where was the sensitivity to what Gary just experienced?* She was a nurse! I tried to suppress the anger that was written on my face.

Before I got in my car, I made the decision that I would agree to the cystoscopy. Neither I nor Gary could go through these catheter changes every six to eight weeks. I made a mental note that I would demand a sedative for the next catheter change. *Why didn't the urologist recommend one?*

Caregiver aloneness is double fold when medical care is needed.

I took Gary to the outpatient cystoscopy a week after our visit with the urologist. The procedure was performed at a regional hospital. I waited for an hour and a half before he was brought into the recovery room. The urologist informed me that he would not operate on Gary.

"It's just not a good option, and I cannot guarantee that putting Gary through this would solve the problem. It might solve the prostate problem, but if the dementia is causing neurological issues that are preventing urine flow, we'll be back to square one."

I was totally deflated. Gary was such a trooper as I attempted to explain to him that the foley needed to stay in place.

I again apologized. "I'm just so sorry, babe. I do not know what to do. Let's go get some lunch. You must be starved."

As we shared lunch, I willed the tears not to flow.

At 7 a.m. the next morning, the facility found Gary on the floor and called EMS. I immediately left for the hospital. Gary was admitted for observation. This would be the fourth hospital stay in eight months. *I prayed the medical staff would have dementia sensitivity.*

When you do this journey alone, there are no hugs, no check-in calls, and no emotional or physical relief. It was 10 p.m. when I left the hospital and reached my car to go home. My physical and emotional tank were empty. I could not remember the last time I had gotten a good night's sleep.

I saw a text message come in from Gary's private nurse. The text was sent in error. "If Gary keeps getting worse, I'll quit. He should be in a nursing home, but Rose is too cheap to put him in one."

I stared into this cruel text. I immediately felt betrayed! *Who does this? How can she say such a thing?* I put the car in gear as another text message came in. It was an apology. She explained, "This stuff happens; it's just a human thing." I let my tears carry me home, hoping I'd be able to fire her soon. *A human thing? There was nothing human in that text!*

Dementia Insensitivity, Inadequate care, the need to advocate.

Gary did not look good when I entered his hospital room the next morning. His head was covered with bandages holding probes in place. They were monitoring brain activity for twelve hours, fearing he might have had a seizure. He was shirtless, and underneath the sheet he wore only a diaper. He appeared heavily sedated and had no food or water for the remainder of the day. I sat with him until 10 p.m. and then returned home.

When I arrived on day three, Gary was still sleeping. I noticed that the bandages and probes had been removed from his head. However, globs of glue remained in his hair. He started to wake up around 11 a.m. I went to the front desk and asked a nurse when a physical therapist would come and evaluate his mobility.

She said, "They have already been here. They said he was unable to walk."

I looked at her. "Surely you jest. How could he possibly get up and walk when he has been fast asleep? Shouldn't they come when he's awake?"

"I don't think they are scheduled to come back," she replied.

I tried to keep my anger in check. "I need to speak to the doctor ASAP. And please get me a comb so I can get the glue out of his hair. Plus, my husband is still without a hospital gown, and he needs changing."

She looked quite annoyed. "I'll get you a comb and check on the other."

I returned to Gary's room, and a comb was delivered. The attending physician and hospital neurologist who visited had no definitive explanation for what had happened two days prior. "We want to keep Gary an additional day until physical therapy can evaluate him."

"I hope they come when he's awake," I replied.

I began combing through his hair, trying to get the glue out. A male nurse entered. Without saying a word, he walked up to Gary's bedside, pulled back the sheet, and began ripping off his diaper. When he reached for his foley catheter with a wet wipe, Gary screamed and swiped at him.

I interrupted, "Excuse me. Can you please talk to my husband before you touch him? You are frightening him. He has later stage dementia."

The nurse's face showed annoyance as he continued to swipe at my husband's penis with a wet wipe. I moved closer to where he stood. Forcing him to acknowledge my presence, I began. "Excuse me. Perhaps you did not hear me. You frighten a dementia patient if you work on him without letting him know what you are doing. Didn't you notice how you startled him? He will understand a kind, gentle voice."

He said, "I have limited time!"

I felt certain he was annoyed he was doing a CNA's job. There were no CNAs assigned to the floor that day.

I said, "I'm sure you do, but you are working on my husband now. Please provide him the respect he deserves."

This was not my first rodeo with a medical professional who had no concept of how to approach and speak with a dementia patient. Without saying a word, the nurse quickly finished what he was doing. As he was leaving Gary's bedside, I said, "Can you please put a gown on my husband and provide an additional blanket? He is cold in only a diaper." He did so and walked out. I stood there in disbelief at what I had witnessed. The nurse had treated Gary as if he were invisible. *How long would Gary have lain like that had I not been there?*

At 7 p.m., after passing a swallow test, Gary's dinner finally arrived. He ate everything. For the first time in three days, he appeared to be returning to baseline, even though he was very unsteady on his feet from lying on his back.

At 8 p.m. a nurse entered the room and checked his IV. She noted that it should be changed. I told her, "The doctor and neurologist said he is permitted to take all medications orally. There is no need for another IV. It will traumatize him." She agreed. Before I left for the night, I went to the nurse's station to make sure she got the order not to insert another IV.

I slept fitfully through the night and arrived emotionally and physically exhausted at 9 a.m. the next day. The first thing I noticed when I entered the room was a new IV inserted. *What?* And Gary was in another deep sleep. *Huh? What happened?*

I marched to the nurse's station and demanded to see the doctor. When he entered the room, I could tell he was uncomfortable. He shifted left to right, and his eyes were downcast.

"WHY was another IV inserted into my husband?" I demanded.

He did not respond.

"I asked you, why was another IV inserted into my husband? You told me that all medication would be given orally. There is nothing even running through that IV!"

He replied, "He kicked a nurse last night."

"That's not what I asked you. I bet he got aggressive when another IV was being inserted! The IV that was not necessary! And what has he been given? Why is he in such a deep sleep?"

The doctor replied, "We gave him Haldol because he was aggressive during the IV change."

I needed to steady myself because I was so furious. It didn't matter how much I advocated, it never seemed to be enough.

"How dare you do that! You had them insert an IV that was unnecessary and gave him Haldol, which over sedates a patient. Gary has had very negative reactions to that medication in the past."

My thoughts went back to the male nurse who had no dementia sensitivity. I could picture Gary sitting in the recliner where I left him the night before, having just eaten, returning to baseline, and smiling. I pictured myself reassuring him and hugging him good night. I could only imagine how frightening it was after I left, when they entered that room and proceeded to insert an IV.

"You're yelling at me," the doctor said.

"I damn well am. I am furious. Why would we all agree on what NOT to do and it's done anyway? You could have called me! I am his POA. I would have come back before you inserted it! You KNOW how traumatic it is for a dementia patient. And it was totally unnecessary! You do not even have fluids running through it. I want his release papers drawn up. There is no reason to keep him here. He didn't have a seizure. It's not definitive he has a UTI. I want him out of here!"

"I'll get it done," he said. "You need to understand, we need to follow protocol."

"Screw your protocol. You need to be more mindful of your patients!"

I sat down. I could feel the tears welling in my eyes. I did not like screaming at anyone. I was at the end of my rope. I looked over at Gary. My heart bled for him. *How much more, God? How much more does this man have to go through?* As much as I tried to protect him, I could not. I felt like I failed him yet again.

He had lost all the progress he had made the day before. Haldol and Gary did not like each other. It would be in his system for days. I felt like my insides were ready to explode. I was frustrated, tired, and angry. The facility would have to agree to take him back, as he would be a fall risk after Haldol. I would also need to hire another sitter to provide 24/7 one-on-one supervision.

Just as I was washing my face of tears, physical therapy came into the room. I looked at them. "Surely you are not going to try and walk my husband now?"

Surely, they tried. I stared in disbelief as they tried to get a drugged man on his feet. They would not clear him as a fall risk because he could not stand, let alone walk. Before they left the room, I asked when they would return. They informed me that hopefully they would be back the next day. No guarantee. I knew I had made the right decision to get him released. I called the facility and explained to the administrator what was going on. She said, "Bring him home. We will do the best we can."

Gary rested throughout the day and when he finally woke a traveling nurse got him cleaned, shaved, and ready for transport. She phoned the kitchen and ordered dinner for both of us. Another angel. She was dementia sensitive and talked while she removed Gary's IV. He didn't even flinch.

We arrived at the facility around 9 p.m. A sitter would begin the next day. Aides were waiting for us and assisted Gary as he walked into the facility. They would change him, put him to bed, and provide 30-minute checks. I vowed before I left the hospital that I would make a full report to the CEO on the lack of care Gary received and the dementia insensitivity that I witnessed. I prayed that Gary would have a good night.

At 11 p.m., shortly after returning home, I got a call that Gary was being transported to another ER closer to the facility. He fell and required stitches. I was certain it was because Haldol was still in his system.

The dementia journey is difficult enough, but when the patient requires medical care, the journey escalates to a whole new level. As strong as I was as a caregiver and skilled as a professional social worker, my strength and skill were diminished during a medical crisis. A nurse verbalized how she felt on an online dementia support group. "I'm a trained nurse with over twenty years of experience. None of my training prepared me for this journey. I've never felt so lost and alone."

Dementia sensitivity and training in all medical environments must be mandated by the medical care commission. Patients should be recognized and not treated as if they were invisible. Caregivers must be listened to and respected. It is imperative that until change takes place, someone with dementia should never be left alone in a hospital or while a medical procedure is being performed.

Call for help

I was very reluctant to dial the number at 11 p.m. I needed help, but I knew the answer would probably be "No." Nonetheless, I would try. The help was for Gary, not me. Perhaps that would make a difference with this family member.

"Hi," I began. "I need some help."

I silently remembered all Gary and I had done for him, financially and otherwise. He, like other family members, had not been present during this journey. He didn't visit Gary or call to check on me.

"What do you need?" I felt hopeful. He lived near the hospital.

"I hate to ask you this, but Gary is in the ER. He had a fall and will require stitches. He just returned to the facility after a week in the hospital. I cannot make the hour and a half drive back there. Can you please stop by the ER and make sure he's alright? He'll be very frightened."

"I'll get back to you," he replied.

"Okay." I breathed a sigh of relief. He probably needed to get changed before he headed out.

Fifteen minutes later I received a text message. It read, *Sorry. I need to be at work at 7 in the morning. I won't be able to stop by.*

I stared at the phone in disbelief. My expectations of those who purported to love Gary dropped to a new low.

Continuing the walk

"Hope is the thing with feathers that perches in the soul
— and sings the tunes without the words —
and never stops at all."

EMILY DICKINSON

Flashback

I had always volunteered, even while working full time and raising a son. Word spreads when you are a willing volunteer, and calls from various agencies found their way to my phone. One day a nonprofit called explaining that a ramp was needed for a boy in a wheelchair who had a rare bone disease. The parents had no funds. They lined up a few guys to build the ramp but had no supplies.

"Would you make some calls and see if you can get anything off our list?" she asked.

"Sure," I replied. "I'll let you know what I'm able to get by the end of the week."

I was able to get all the supplies needed from local businesses. The generosity of people always surprised me. All you had to do was ask. I called the agency on Friday with the wonderful news only to learn their disappointing news. The guys who had committed to the project could not do it. I got the address where the ramp was needed and told them I'd see what I could do.

Gary (my handy dandy man) walked into the house late that night. He was returning from a weeklong business trip. I was in our bedroom reading, and as soon as he looked at my face he knew something was wrong.

"What's up?"

I explained the situation to him.

Without skipping a beat, he said, "I'll call my friends tomorrow. When do they want it done?"

"Tomorrow," I replied.

"Don't worry about it. Go to sleep. I'll set my alarm. We'll get it done."

And he did. Because that's who Gary was.

July 4, 2021

- 27 years ago, Steve came into our home.
- 21 years ago, we moved to North Carolina.
- 15 years ago, we moved from the mountains to the North Carolina coast.
- 7 years ago, we moved back to the mountains.
- All on July 4.

All memory markers.

The sidewalks and streets were jammed with tourists in our small town. I had a difficult time navigating Gary and myself to our familiar haunts. I was determined to make it a great day, so I found a beautiful walk area around the Tuckasegee River. When I arrived at the pull-off point, Gary was already tired, so we sat with Chase beside us, enjoying the sun and warm weather. I had purchased some milkshakes beforehand, and Gary eagerly took his and began to drink.

I handed him a sandwich. His memory failed him as he stared at it, not quite sure what to do. I picked mine up and demonstrated how to hold it "Just eat it like this," I instructed. He smiled as he said, "Thanks, Mom."

I joked with him. "Okay, so now I'm your mom?" He laughed. "You are still a pain in my butt," I said. He laughed harder. It was far better for us to laugh than cry. There was no stopping this insidious disease.

Memories flashed in and out of my mind throughout the day. I glanced over at Gary and remembered how he once was. I wanted so much to have him back, if only for a few minutes. I forced myself not to be sad.

I counted the years. Ten years since I first noticed that something was wrong with Gary. Seven years since I grew determined to find out what was wrong. Three years since he was given a dementia diagnosis.

Continuing the walk

I stopped at Food Lion on the way back. As we exited, I waited patiently as Gary's steps were so slow.

"It's okay, babe. Take your time."

A younger man walked by.

He smiled as he said, "I hope when I'm an old man I have a sweetie that will call me babe."

It made my day and allowed me to enjoy a smile.

We returned to his room at the facility. As I prepared to leave, I reassured Gary that I'd call that night. "I'll see you in a couple days," I said as I reached for a hug.

"Thank you," he replied. "I really appreciate what you do. You're so nice."

"I've got your back, babe. I always will. Even when you no longer know I am here, I will be."

"Thank you," he said. "What's your name again?"

Sometimes it just feels good to laugh.

My mood matched the threatening gray clouds. I fought unhappiness. Every visit was a reminder of dementia stealing one more thing from Gary. To help counteract the gloom, I began to count my blessings. I concentrated on Gary becoming stable after months of UTIs, hospitalizations, and ER visits. I imagined myself going on a day trip filled with laughter and joy. I thought of anything I could to wash the frown from my face before I entered the facility. It wasn't a gift I wished to bring him.

I put a smile on my face before walking into his room. He and I walked down to the dining room. I sat across from him as he ate. I offered help when he tried to cut his sandwich with a spoon.

"Here, let me cut it for you."

As we drove away from the facility, I noted his increased confusion as he tried to navigate the world around him.

"What's that?" he asked when a car passed with a loud muffler..

"What's that?" he asked when I opened the car window.

"What's that?" he asked when the car beeped because I switched lanes.

"What's that?" he asked when I turned on my blinker.

I made sure he didn't see my eyes roll. I pushed away my guilt from just feeling tired of it all. I consoled myself, *It's okay, Rose. You're only human.*

I took him on his favorite walk at the Grist Mill in Smoky National Park. Being in nature calmed my soul and spirit, and I felt a sense of peace envelop him. Gary always loved being outdoors. The clouds started to disperse, carrying away the gloom, and the sun peeked out. I enjoyed its warmth wrapping its arms around us.

I saw a woman, my guess a daughter, assisting her much older father, who was using a cane for support. Her mother, who walked behind them, struggled in a leg brace, pushing a walker. As Gary and

I navigated the dirt path around them, I whispered, "Well, we finally found others who are slower than you."

And in that moment, we broke into spontaneous laughter. Gripping our stomachs, we looked at each other with tears rolling down our faces. We must have looked like idiots to those who passed us, but we did not care. It was laughter that only we understood. It's those moments on a dementia journey that you hold onto for dear life.

September 2021

Follow your gut.

The administrator at the facility told me that she had found a hospice agency that would monitor and care for Gary's catheter. That was such great news! I fired his private nurse. My hurt was still raw from the text she misdirected at me.

Gary was scheduled to have his catheter changed. I decided that I wanted the catheter left out to see if Gary could urinate on his own. The urologist had doubts that Gary would be successful but felt no damage would be done if it was left out for ten hours. Hospice felt comfortable with six hours, so I compromised on eight.

I was about to lose my mind with worry when at the seventh hour I received a call that Gary urinated! Everyone was elated. I pushed back any dread that his ability to void enough urine would not last. I had my first good night's sleep in months, without the fear that he was going to pull out his foley and cause damage. Gary was taking methenamine to prevent future UTIs. I kept my fingers and toes crossed that his urinary tract would stay healthy.

As the month ended, I received the sad news that the administrator of the facility would be leaving. She was such a huge advocate for Gary and a support to me. I also received news that six residents tested positive for Covid. It appeared as soon as one cause for anxiety went away, it was replaced with another.

What tool can I find to keep Gary occupied?

I was worried about the endless hours Gary sat idle. I searched for things that might occupy his time or entertain him. Even though his short-term memory was less than five minutes, I continued to try to teach him things. The resolve in me kept burning despite countless failures because I loved him, and I wanted this journey to be easier.

I found a neon orange stress ball and decided to purchase it. I convinced myself that this was something that Gary could sit with, squeeze, and playfully witness the many shapes that it would produce. I also felt it might alleviate his recent anxiety. Along with that purchase, I found a unique, colorful plastic bird. If you held out your fingertip, it would remain balanced there.

I instructed Gary to hold out his finger. He held out his arm hand side down. I gently instructed, "Watch me. Extend your arm, palm side up, finger extended." He tried but did the same as before. I gently turned his hand over and extended one finger. The bird stayed balanced on it, but Gary got afraid. He grabbed it with the other hand, convinced it would crash to the ground. "I don't want to hurt the bird!" he shouted, frightened.

Not wanting to give up, I gave Gary ample time to watch as I demonstrated what could be done with the stress ball. It appeared he understood, so I handed it to him. Within half a second, he lifted it to his mouth to bite into it. *He thinks it's an orange!* I was in utter disbelief and took it from him.

I resigned myself to the fact that at this stage of dementia Gary was not able to process enough for me to introduce him to new things.

A Visit to My Sister-in-Law's

My widowed sister-in-law lived fifteen minutes from the facility, so, when I picked Gary up for an outing, my car inevitably headed in her direction. My brother had passed away from a heart attack eleven years prior. She and my brother were two of the reasons Gary and I relocated to North Carolina in 2000.

Christi had a dog, and he and Chase were good friends. So, while we sat and talked, watched TV, or had a snack, Chase had an afternoon to run and play in Christi's yard. Christi provided unlimited support to me with her great listening ears and offered to watch Chase at any hour of the day or night. If Gary had an ER visit or hospitalization, she would meet me there and take Chase home with her rather than have him stay at the facility.

She always welcomed us in her home and was very patient with Gary, even when he spoke gibberish. She never hesitated to try and engage with him. She'd set up a tray table, bring him his favorite drink, and make him feel safe and at home.

When we arrived for a visit, Gary was struggling with a bad stomach. I followed him into the bathroom. If I did not, I'd find him wandering in another room. Gary had difficulty getting his athletic pants down and navigating the pull up. Also, this toilet was lower than those in the facility, and there was no grab bar. Any change to the environment made it difficult for him to adjust. As he attempted to sit down, he screamed, fearing he'd fall into the toilet.

"No, no, no" he whimpered, his voice trembling with fear.

"It's okay, babe, I've got his. I won't let you fall." I'd reassure him.

He was experiencing loose bowel movements, so I sat on the edge of her tub and comforted him. He could not process why his bowels were different today. It frightened him because he no longer understood when his body was behaving differently.

When he was done, I handed him toilet paper. His hand had such a tremor that I knew he had not sufficiently wiped himself. I pulled over a standalone cabinet so he'd have something to hold onto and helped him rise from the seat. I was mortified that his rear end was covered with loose bowels. I held my breath. The stench was so bad.

I knew I had to clean him. There were many things I did and witnessed with Gary, but this was the first time I would need to clean his butt. It almost felt unnatural to do this to a grown man. And even stranger for me was the fact that Gary did not protest. A few years earlier he would have been mortified. *Later, changing or cleaning private parts would produce aggression. It happens with nearly all dementia patients. Dementia does not steal the instinct for modesty and taking care of one's toileting.*

I began running warm water, opened Christi's linen closet, and literally used every one of her washcloths to clean him. I simply could not stand my hands on the stained washcloths. I had changed many babies' diapers, but somehow this felt different to me. Witnessing an educated grown man who had traveled the world regress is very difficult. Once he was clean, I returned him to the living room.

Christi never mentioned her laundry basket filled with soiled washcloths. I vaguely remembered half mentioning it to her, but she shrugged it off. She always showed grace interacting with Gary's illness and my position as his caregiver. While she may have been tempted, she never offered advice, an opinion, or criticism. What she did provide was endless listening, love, and support. I will always be grateful for that.

Shake Your Booty

As I settled in for an hour and a half ride to the facility, I immediately felt frustrated as I ticked off all the things left undone at home. However, I pushed my frustration aside. Today I would concentrate on Gary. I decided to treat him to lunch. As we settled into our seats at a nearby restaurant, I looked over at him.

"Okay, so what's my name?"

He smiled back. "I know, but I can't remember."

"Multiple choice. Rose, Linda, or Sally?"

He looked puzzled, then responded, "Rose?"

I reached over and gave him a high five.

He looked upward and whispered, "Thank you, God."

I laughed. "Whatcha afraid of? That I'll kick your butt if you don't remember my name?"

He laughed. Dementia usually steals a person's personality, but Gary's sense of humor was still intact.

After lunch we headed to the park for a walk. I noted that I had slowed my walk to a crawl, and yet Gary still lagged two feet behind. A song stirred in my head, and I began to dance, unperturbed by others walking in the park. I circled back and danced around Gary.

He started to laugh, his blue eyes crinkling up at the sides.

"Come on, old man, shake your booty."

He continued to laugh and shook his butt.

When he arrived back at the facility, the stress from the outing drained from his face. He was back in his safe zone. The staff greeted and welcomed him home, as they always did. In his room he gravitated toward the couch. I gave him chocolate milk and an oatmeal raisin cookie I had purchased at the restaurant. They were his favorites. I kissed our dog goodbye and headed to my car. Today was a good day.

I rolled the windows halfway down, powered on the radio, and listed to the tunes of soul town. I cranked it up. I sank into my seat and let the music reach into every cell of my being, washing away my anticipatory grief and the stress of watching a man I loved decline.

Diana Ross's voice boomed over the radio. "*Reach out and touch somebody's hand. Make this world a better place if you can.*" My mind danced to the music all the way home.

Respite

I escaped for five days. I felt if I did not get a break that I would get sick and explode into a million hurtful pieces. Many in-home caregivers never have the luxury of respite. So, I felt blessed for the opportunity. At the same time, it was hard to begin a vacation anxiety-ridden and drained. I found myself searching for energy just to get a suitcase packed. My mind was so foggy and confused that I needed to write a list of how much underwear, pants, shirts, etc., to pack.

Ralph agreed to come while I was away and make a business trip out of it. He would work in a nearby hotel but could visit his dad at lunch and dinner. It was important that someone be nearby at all times, as Gary's disease was progressing, and emergency calls were happening more frequently.

I decided to visit with two friends. One was having a large celebration for her son. The other friend had taken a fall four years prior and was paralyzed. Since Gary's diagnosis I had been unable to visit her. I notified my nieces a month in advance that I would be in the area and would love to meet them for lunch or dinner, but both were busy. I was disappointed, as they were like daughters to Gary and me, and I had no idea when I'd have another opportunity to travel.

The celebration my friend hosted for her son was beautiful. It was much bigger than I had anticipated, with nearly a hundred guests. My bestie of over thirty years and her family opened their hearts and home to me. "Just try to relax. Eat. Have some fun," they told me. "Our home is your home."

Nearing the end of her son's birthday/graduation/off to college celebration, his dad got up to speak. He shared in detail parts of his son's childhood and the times they shared together. You could hear the pride in his voice as he spoke of his son's accomplishments and his acceptance into Syracuse University. When his dad finished, his son got up to speak. He spoke of the gratitude and love he had for his parents. He finished by crediting his parents with so much of who he was.

I tried hard to hold back tears as memories of Gary and our life with our sons flooded my mind. It seemed like yesterday that Steve left for college. I remembered my happiness as I had settled him into his college dorm and the joy I felt when he returned home with all his friends. One time Gary and I hosted his entire baseball team at a nearby recreation center. Equal memories of times shared with Gary's son and his family flooded my mind. The sad reality was Gary and I had not seen Steve for three years, and we rarely spoke. Since his dad's diagnosis any attempt at conversation failed.

Families can be messy, but I missed mine. I had felt the absence since diagnosis from siblings, nieces, nephews, daughters-in-laws, grandchildren, and sons in whom Gary and I had invested time and love. I grieved that soon Gary would be gone, and he would not have a chance to feel their love or say goodbye. I also missed the opportunity to share time, meals, and conversation with them. So much time had already passed. *What were they waiting for?*

I exited the party and retreated to my room because my sadness was overwhelming. I did not want to spoil the special day for such good friends of mine. I finished the week with my other friend in New Hampshire. She and her husband opened their home and went out of their way to make me feel loved and cared for. Near the end of five days, just as I was beginning to relax, I needed to return home.

As the plane touched down, calls and text messages started coming in from the facility. "Gary is doing okay. But Chase keeps escaping from his room. You need to take him home with you. He can no longer stay with Gary. Please call ASAP."

I added a dog to my list of responsibilities.

Timeline of Loss

When I attended preadoption workshops, the instructor asked each of us to make a list of everything and everyone that was important in our life. And then she told us, "Starting at the most important, go down the list and cross off each one, one by one." When our lists were all crossed off, she told us, "That is what it's like when a child enters the foster system. They enter a home losing everyone and everything they knew. And each of those losses is a trauma event."

I feel dementia can be described as such. And it's not just the patient who suffers. The trauma extends to the caregiver. The patient feels the loss as it occurs; then it is forgotten. But the empathetic caregiver feels the loss and retains the memory.

Gary's journey was a timeline of loss. And the list kept growing. Returning from my trip, I needed to prepare him to say goodbye to his dog. Chase entered assisted living with him and had been his salvation. The facility went above and beyond to care for him so he and Gary would not be separated. But the facility could no longer risk the safety of the other residents. Chase was sneaking out of the room and running down the hallways. They feared he might run into a resident and cause a fall.

The administrator put a lot of thought into her decision. She assured me that the time was right. Gary was not mindful of having the dog anymore. Still, it pained me to have to separate them. I asked her for a week to gather my thoughts. I found a robotic dog on Amazon and ordered it. When it arrived, I noted how lifelike it was and prayed that it would provide some comfort to Gary.

Before I arrived at the facility, I had Chase's belongings brought to the front of the building. I loaded them into the back of the car. I then found Gary in the dining room. After he finished eating, he and Chase accompanied me to the car.

I sat beside Gary and held his hand. "Babe, concentrate. I need you to understand me."

"Okay." he said. I was never sure if he would, but I asked anyway.

I began. "I *really* need Chase to stay with me. I miss him so much. Please, just for a few days. I promise to take good care of him and will bring him to visit. Is that okay?"

He hesitated. With pleading in his voice, he said, "Will I still see him?"

"Of course, sweetheart. I will bring him to visit you all the time. I promise. You know I keep my promises."

"Okay," he replied. I'm not sure he understood what I was asking, but he trusted me. Every type of dementia is different, and everyone responds differently to it. I was blessed that inherently Gary knew I always had his best interests at heart. I'm not sure where in the abyss his memories went to rest and why certain ones remained outside. I was just grateful that his trust in me remained.

When we got back to the facility, I introduced him to the robotic dog. Gary looked at me. "Is it real?" he asked.

"It's as real as you want it to be," I replied.

I was learning to meet Gary where he was and not where I was in accepting his disease. The administrator was right. Gary suffered no ill effects from Chase being gone, but I made sure to bring him on every visit.

When I did visit with the dog, Gary would pet him and say, "Hi, buddy," and that was it. Gary got used to the robotic dog, and I occasionally found the dog's neck wet from where he attempted to give him a drink. Although Gary's emotions appeared unharmed, I fought daily to keep mine under control.

Get those feet back in the car

I believe if the Lord wanted us to look back, he'd make the rearview mirror larger than the front windshield of our car. Today as I drove Gary back to the facility after an outing, I couldn't help but look back to happier times.

I remembered myself twenty years earlier riding in the passenger seat with legs outstretched on the dash. My bare feet hanging out the car window with the wind whipping through my toes.

"Ya better get those feet back in the car," Gary said, laughing.

I looked at him, "Drive, master, drive." I felt the freedom from the high heels and business suits that were my standard garb when I navigated a career in IT. Two whole weeks of just living lay ahead of us.

We took road trips often. We'd just get in the car and drive wherever we wanted. On this trip, we were heading to Sarasota, Florida. We'd spend a few days with friends and then take off for new adventures. We had our snorkeling equipment in the car and looked forward to time in the ocean. I looked over at him and asked, "Do you realize we have not spoken to each other in five hours?" He smiled and winked at me, "We don't have to." We always felt so comfortable with each other whether in silence or sharing our innermost thoughts.

I returned to reality as I pulled into the facility, gathering goodies I purchased for Gary. Mini chocolate milks, snacks, and a caramel sundae. After getting him settled in his room and giving him a hug, I said, "I'll see you in a couple days."

Smiling he said, "Thank you. I'm sorry. What's your name again?"

"My name is Rose."

No matter how many times Gary forgot my name, it always felt like the first time. The jarring realization that my husband did not know my name shook my soul to its core. Hearing someone say your name is personal. It has a psychological effect. It makes you feel valued, remembered, and seen.

Throughout the journey, the hurt of his not knowing me by my name, or especially "babe," made me feel not valued as his wife, his lifelong companion. Rather it felt like I was a stranger playing a role with no reciprocation of emotion or love. It was so odd that although Gary didn't know my name, he never failed to let me know he loved me. That helped, but his not knowing my name unintentionally hurt an already shattered heart.

Trying to recapture joy

Gary was always an outdoorsman. The hills were alive with color that fall. I decided to treat him for a ride on the Blue Ridge Parkway. There were many lookout points to view the colorful mountain ranges.

Gary was sleepy and a bit more confused than usual when I picked him up. I hit the button for the sunroof in my car. I hoped that the fresh air would help wake him up. I anticipated the joy I would feel when Gary saw the mountains ranges that he loved so much.

I guided him out of the car at the first turnoff. He was no longer able to navigate on his own. It appeared he forgot how. *When did that happen?* I pointed his eyes in the direction of the mountain range. But he kept looking toward the road. *Why is he doing that?*

"No, this way." I prompted. "Look this way."

But his mind was confused. It whispered to me, *I don't know what to do. What am I supposed to do?*

He turned around and began to aimlessly walk down the path toward the parking lot. I tried prompting him back, because he was missing all the fun. I let him walk and followed him. At the next lookout point, it was much the same. Conceding that he wasn't enjoying the views, I found a picnic table and laid out our lunch. The bees were busy keeping us company, and I spent my time shooing them away so that Gary could enjoy his sandwich. But he wasn't hungry and barely ate. I threw the rest away, and we headed back to the car.

I tried not to let the disappointment affect me, but my heart was sobbing. Try as I might, I could not recapture any of the fun we once shared. I felt bad for Gary and bad for myself. I felt I had so little joy in my life. I would never again experience the man with whom I shared so much. Gary slept all the way home, while I had only my thoughts to keep me company.

When we returned, a resident asked, "Can you check on Eve? She hasn't been out of her room all day."

As I entered Eve's room, she greeted me warmly.

"Hi, dear," she said, "Are you visiting me?"

"Yes. Is something wrong?" I asked. "Your friends are worried about you."

"No, dear, I'm just a bit down today."

"I'm sorry," I said. "I understand." I told her about my day. "I wonder if this is all that the Lord has left for me."

Her face lit up. "No, dear, the Lord has wonderful things planned for you. Something you can't even imagine."

She pointed her finger down. "He brings you down to the valley." And then with a huge smile, she pointed her finger up. "And then he brings you up. Higher than you can ever imagine."

I reached over and gave her a huge hug. "Thank you," I said. "I needed that."

I left the facility with my spirit renewed.

December 2021

A lot of staff had left the facility since new management took over. I began feeling uncomfortable, because the trust in staff I spent years developing no longer existed.

I stocked Gary's room with drinks and noticed many remained untouched. His toilet seat was loose, and it took over a week with multiple reminders to get it screwed on tightly. His room was dirty, and I noticed gnats on his wall. There were no waste bags in his garbage cans, and the paper towel dispenser in his bathroom was always empty. I found wet spills covering his floor on one visit. Brand new slippers and shoes were missing, as was a wreath that hung on his door. Snacks that I replenished and kept in the room couldn't be found. And a holiday gift card I left for Gary's main caregiver was stolen.

I found myself cleaning his room every time I visited. I filed weekly reports, but I always found the room in the same condition. I continued to press the new administrator for answers, but he never followed up. I was becoming more and more uneasy.

I was also seeing changes in Gary that warned me his dementia was progressing. He was very sensitive to touch. He would jump and scream if I touched his skin. If he was in a room with people talking, he'd get visibly agitated. It appeared to be too much stimulation. When I visited or took him out, he could barely sit still.

He needed constant prompting to drink. If I handed him a drink, he'd ask, "What's this?" If I took him out to eat, he would doze off with a mouthful of food. He was urinating everywhere in the facility, and one day he defecated in the courtyard. At different times throughout the day, he would bang on residents' doors. A few times he went to the front door and shook the exit bar, wanting to get out. And he was getting aggressive with residents. He pushed one resident, but the staff intervened so the resident was not injured. Gary also experienced a seizure in the dining room, and staff reported he stopped breathing and turned blue. By the time EMS got there, he was okay. I was in frequent touch with the care manager, but I could never establish a time to speak with the new administrator about how we were going to handle the advancement of Gary's disease.

The care manager and I revised his care plan, establishing a new routine for a.m. and p.m. We cut down his intake of sugary snacks, increased hydration, and made sure Gary was brought outside for fresh air during the day. The television was to be left on only during the day. Our attempt to get him into a routine was intended to help with the sundowning he was experiencing.

Sundowning is a term used with dementia to describe a state of confusion that often occurs in the late afternoon and spans into the night. In addition to confusion, there are a variety of behaviors, such as aggression, anxiety, rummaging through things, and wandering. The facility doctor felt Gary had enough cognition to be redirected when he wandered. But the night staff disagreed.

The doctor's suggestion of Ativan, a tranquilizer to discourage anxiety and induce sleep, did not work. The doctor then tried Trazodone. She hoped this medication would regulate serotonin and influence sleep. 50 mg put Gary in a stupor, and the staff feared it would increase his fall risk, so it was discontinued.

I was exhausted from the constant calls from the facility. Challenges were occurring daily with no resolution. I phoned the administrator again and requested a meeting. I explained I needed to get consistent reports of what was happening with Gary, and we needed a new game plan. He promised to get all the staff together, talk to them, and get back to me. He never did. I followed up with text messages. Still no response. When I visited the facility, he was nowhere to be found. My frustration and concerns were mounting daily, along with my worries about Gary. His safety net was developing new holes every day.

Transitioning Gary frightened me, as I was aware of transfer trauma. A new location would influence his psychological well-being, mood, and behavior. I also feared all the work it involved. Transitioning would involve tons of paperwork, notifying insurance, visiting facilities, interviewing, and again familiarizing myself with all new staff. I gathered my strength and moved forward looking for a memory care placement that could provide more one-on-one supervision.

Gary's symptoms — 2021

Late-stage dementia — 3.5 years since diagnosis

- Gary is having problems getting off the toilet. If there is no toilet paper on the roll, he will use his hands.
- He is rummaging through his things all the time.
- He carries a lot of his belongings from his room.
- He calls 911 frequently, so most of the numbers on his phone are duct taped.
- He will disconnect his phone and push his chair down the hall.
- He wanders throughout the night and bangs on people's doors.
- He is taking off all his clothes with no modesty.
- He sleeps most of the day.
- He is very sensitive to touch.
- He is easily agitated in a room full of people.
- He goes into the dining room frequently looking for food.
- He can rarely articulate a full sentence.
- He calls at random times throughout the day and night talking gibberish.
- He is urinating everywhere and defecating in the courtyard.
- He is aggressive during sundowning.
- All his medications are crushed into pudding or applesauce.

His heart knows me, and he always expresses gratitude.

Dementia caregivers

Previously, I talked about people having a sensitivity trait to other people's suffering. Those are the *can-do caregivers*. They can and will do everything to provide and care for someone they love. No one needs to ask them to do anything. They are ten steps ahead, insuring their loved one's well-being.

There's another group of people. They are the *want-to-do*. They want to do what they can when it's convenient. They are the ones who will have a reason why they can't be a *can-do caregiver*. I live too far away. I have my own family. It stresses me out. I want to remember how they were before. I can't take family leave. This is the larger group of people. These are the ones the *can-do* caregivers expect help and support from. It's a fight that the *can-do caregiver* will not win. It's a difficult fact to reconcile.

Dementia caregivers who have had difficulties receiving help shared what they would have done differently. They would have accepted that in discussions with some they'd never be right. They should have taken advice with a grain of salt. They would not have attended to every argument and should have allowed the other person to be wrong. They should have accepted that not everyone was like them. They would make it clear that you cannot walk away and then give opinions and criticize. They would have told the few who sent flowers and offered prayers that, while they are nice things to do, supporting and helping are better.

I respect that everyone is busy with their own responsibilities, but picking up a phone, offering support to both patient and caregiver, sending a card or small gift to the patient on a holiday, and making visits to show your love and demonstrate a bit of humanity is not a lot to ask. Especially to those who have loved and supported you.

I was entering the last chapter of Gary's life, and I knew it would be the roughest stage of dementia. Late-stage dementia takes a huge amount of energy, effort, and love, whether in a facility or at home.

There is no shame in admitting that one needs help with facility care. This stage demands a village. Often the in-home caregiver will begin to break at this point. The mopping up of urine and feces, the incontinence and changing of diapers, the patient being awake during the night, and the aggressiveness that follows late-stage dementia contributes to caregiver exhaustion and stress. Constantly coaxing a loved one to eat and drink, authorizing medications that sometimes produce nasty side effects, and watching material things being destroyed take a mental toll. Seeing a loved one wheelchair or bedbound, nonverbal, plagued by bedsores, and generally deteriorating will exhaust any caregiver. It's a lot of suffering to witness and process while retaining your sensibilities to take care of someone.

Unfortunately, for many in-home caregivers there is no money for a facility or in-home care. Many patients are not eligible for Medicaid, and outside care is extremely expensive. Assets by late stage are usually depleted. Even if a facility is found, there are waiting lists, and the loved one needs to pass an assessment. Many facilities will not accept a patient who demonstrates a lot of the behaviors seen with this stage of dementia. If family were not around before, they most certainly wouldn't be now. The worn and weary caregiver who has provided care for so many years begins to crumble.

As you will see in the next section, even facility care becomes a huge issue. Our society sadly throws people away who are in need. Money isn't the only challenge. Caregivers quickly find out the difference between competent and incompetent staff.

It is critical in this stage that the caregiver practices some form of self-care. It could be taking a walk or bath, talking with a friend, stepping outside for a breath of fresh air, eating healthy foods, or exercising.

I was prepared to persevere and get to the other side of dementia. There was no time to regurgitate the anger and hurt I felt previously or entertain self-pity in any form. Whatever strength I had left, I would share it with Gary. Together we would weather the last storms of his life.

Entering late stage

"The tragedy of life is what dies inside a man while he lives."

ALBERT SCHWEITZER

January 2022
Picking a new facility

By January 2, Gary had lost ten pounds, although he still had a healthy appetite. I knew a ten-pound drop was a criterion to get hospice back on board. I welcomed it. It would give me another set of eyes at the facility. I asked hospice if they had a volunteer who could visit Gary.

I was surprised to receive a call almost immediately from Linda. She had recently moved to the area. Linda was a retired police officer and had recently become a hospice volunteer. She was delighted to help. I remember standing in my kitchen after the call came in and crying from the sheer joy of having someone's help. After discussing with her my observations at the facility, she agreed to keep a close eye on things and report back to me.

Hospice was now giving Gary his showers because of the length of time it took. Many dementia patients are frightened by water hitting their head, and, because they are always cold, they dread the shower. Hospice had the time to spend with Gary. They would crank the room up past 80 degrees and use a shower wand to clean him instead of putting him under a shower head. It took a long time to undress and instruct Gary in the shower. One day after bathing him, the hospice nurse reported that when she walked in his room, she found Gary urine-soaked on his futon. She immediately reported it to the care manager. I was very grateful to have hospice on board who provided another set of eyes.

I made a half dozen calls to memory care facilities. No one answered, so I left messages. I received no calls back. The two I did manage to reach had six month waiting lists and were $5,000 more a month. I read an article about a newly renovated memory care facility and was pleased to learn it was only twenty-five minutes from my home. I scheduled a visit.

It was a much smaller facility and appeared comfy, cozy, and clean. I was assured of many things, including little staff turnover and staff that were fully trained and experienced. These were important criteria to me in choosing a facility. The administrator agreed to visit Gary at his present assisted living facility. She would meet with the care manager and administrator, gather all his information, and let me know if they'd accept him.

During that time, I called the local ombudsman and got a very favorable review of this facility. She told me, "This facility is run well. I know them personally." I checked online reviews from caregivers, and I checked the DHHS site for infractions. I made several visits at different times, and each time I liked what I saw. I did not see any red flags. They had a more structured schedule for the residents, and the food was a step up from the facility he was leaving. Memory care was priced at $6,200 a month, an almost $2,700 increase. At that rate, Gary's long-term benefits would end sooner. Medication management, cable TV, toiletries, and pull-ups were not covered in that cost.

I phoned his facility and let the staff know that Gary would be transitioning in February. I notified Ralph that I would need help with the transition. I asked him to stay longer than a few days, but he committed to four days. Communication with Steve was still strained or nonexistent. Even though he offered to help during a recent brief call, I did not feel I could summarize years' worth of care. He had not received a Covid vaccine, and I could not afford to have him show up and infect his dad and other residents.

Entering late stage

February 2022

I spent a week packing up Gary's belongings and getting rid of clothes, etc., that were no longer being used. I'm not sure Gary understood what transitioning meant, but while packing his things I would rave about the wonderful place he'd be living. I'd share that it was much closer to my home, and I'd be able to see him more often. He did not appear upset with the prospect of the move.

On the morning of the move, I met Ralph at the facility. While he loaded Gary's belongings into his rental car, I helped Gary remain calm. I felt myself go numb as his room was being emptied. This had been his home for three and a half years! My stomach churned with anticipation. How would Gary be affected by this transition? I was happy, sad, and scared to death at the same time. I found a smile and plastered it on my face. I was puzzled why the administrator and many of the staff did not take the time to say goodbye and wish Gary well.

When we arrived at the new facility, I got busy setting up his room. His son helped a great deal and was given the task of labeling new clothes. The care manager and medical technician came in and introduced themselves. Although I was apprehensive when I left that evening, I felt I had made the right choice.

For the next two days, Ralph and I visited Gary. Many facilities tell the family to stay away for a while to give the resident time to settle in. We were not told that. I was led to believe that anything we could do to ease the transition would be worthwhile. In retrospect, providing time to adjust is the better choice.

I found these visits more difficult. The routine was different from assisted living, and all the residents had later stage dementia. Without the non-dementia residents whose company I had enjoyed at assisted living, I felt overwhelmingly sad that this was a new normal for Gary.

Gary appeared to be weathering the transition well enough, but I was concerned, as he was still without adequate medication. I knew his aggressiveness would kick in soon. I mentioned it several times to staff, but everyone was waiting on others' schedules so that a team meeting could be held.

An hour after Ralph arrived home, I received a call from the facility. Gary had become aggressive and threw furniture across the dayroom. He was sedated with Haldol. I was furious and put a call into the facility's primary physician. She assured me that it was a low dose. I told her, "Gary will not do well on that drug!" It was a Friday evening. She told me, "It's the only tool in our toolbox. We'll continue it until a team meeting on Monday."

I tried to relax, but when I saw Gary on Saturday, I was alarmed. He appeared zombie-like. By Sunday evening, he had suffered a seizure. Hospice was onboard, so he was not transported to the ER. There was nothing to be done except let him sleep it off. I spent Monday through Wednesday at his bedside until he woke up and returned to baseline. I was upset with Ralph because I was alone again to handle a crisis.

I was not pleased that the team meeting took place nearly two weeks later and that the only medication Gary was given for his aggression was Ativan. I was riddled with anxiety that this placement would disrupt, and Gary would have nowhere to go. A stop order was put on Haldol, and it was added to his allergy list.

When we met as a team, it was decided to try Gary on a low dose of Seroquel and increase it every second week until an optimum dosage was reached. The hope was that it would curb his aggression. Trazodone would be given at night to induce sleep, and Ativan would be pulled slowly, as they felt it was working in reverse and increasing his agitation. The care manager felt that working with Gary on redirection, using a different tone of voice, and providing one-on-one supervision would help in curbing the aggression.

Gary's aggression continued, so I suggested a log be implemented so that triggers could be identified. However, none were. After seven weeks, I was assured by the care manager that Gary was doing much better. One medical technician shared, "We hit the magic number, Rose. Smooth sailing from here on out. Gary is doing great!"

However, I began noticing red flags at the facility. Gary's hygiene was not good. I found him unshaven and in urine-soaked pull-ups more than once. Items disappeared from his room, and the facility was short-staffed on weekends. I also noted attitudes among the staff. I mentioned the staffing issue to the administrator. I was assured that they were trying to correct the problem. Still, I was not happy. I was told before transitioning Gary that they had adequate coverage and no turnover.

I was also concerned that residents were corralled into one room and monitored by cameras from the office. Sometimes no staff were in that room. Residents had little interaction with staff and were not taken outside on nice days. I thought Gary would receive more one-on-one time.

During this transition, I learned Steve was in town. He told me he'd be visiting his dad for four days. He had been absent for some time, so I was happy that he made the time to see his father. However, he made no time to visit me. He opted to stay at a hotel where he would be closer to his friends.

I vowed to stay on top of things at the facility so that Gary would not have to experience another transfer trauma. I met with the administrator, and we had a meeting of the minds. She promised to address my issues regarding Gary's care.

March 2022

Within a reasonable time frame, all my concerns were addressed. I continued to call daily and visit two or three times a week. I was building a good rapport with the staff, and so was Linda. Hospice allowed her to volunteer at the new facility. I was grateful Linda agreed as her driving time was increased. I questioned the care manager about Gary's aggression, and she gave a favorable report. "I've been working every night. I haven't seen any problems. I feel he's doing great!"

My visits with Gary began at lunchtime so I could observe what he ate. I noted the food was freshly prepared and healthier than at assisted living. He still had a good appetite. We would then head outside the facility. I'd stop at Dunkin' Donuts for his favorite mocha frappe and an apple spice donut (his favorite) and then direct my car to a nearby lake.

On one visit, I suggested we go to Big Lots. He immediately agreed and said, "Sure." I was very surprised that he not only comprehended what I said but that he wasn't as antsy. The medications were working! As we passed the Easter decorations, he pointed at a large glass egg and said, "I like that." I smiled. I had purchased that same egg for my home a few weeks before. For a moment, I had Gary back. When it came to buying things in our home, we always shared the same taste.

I returned him to the facility as the shift was changing. I always tried to return him later so I could speak with the night shift coming on. An aide came up to us.

"Welcome home, Gary! Did you have a nice time?"

Gary smiled.

"We had a wonderful time!" I replied.

The aide gave him a hug. She smiled at me and said, "He is the best resident we have. He's so sweet. He walks down the halls blowing kisses at everyone."

I felt relieved that day when I left the facility. I was so happy he had settled in; my concerns had been addressed and he was now properly medicated. Little did I know this was the last outing Gary and I would share. It still breaks my heart as I recollect this memory.

Eviction notice

"Ask no questions and you'll hear no lies."

JAMES JOYCE

Fear

It is said that before entering the sea
A river trembles with fear.
She looks back at the path she has traveled,
from the peaks of the mountains,
the long winding road crossing forests and villages.
And in front of her,
She sees an ocean so vast,
that to enter
there seems nothing more to disappear forever.
But there is no other way,
The river can not go back.
Nobody can go back.
To go back is impossible in existence.
The river needs to take the risk
of entering the ocean
because only than will fear disappear,
because that's where the river will know
it's not about disappearing in the ocean,
but of becoming the ocean.

BY KHALIL GIBRAN

End of March 2022

I reached for the phone and dialed the facility. I inquired how Gary was doing, as I had done every day.

"Wonderful. For the most part he is doing great," the med tech reported. "We had an episode last night, but we handled it."

"Okay," I said. "I'll check back with you tomorrow. I'll be there in a day or two for a visit. Give Gary a big hug for me."

"Will do. Have a great day, Rose. Relax, everything is going well." I hung up the phone smiling.

A moment later the phone rang. I thought, *they must have forgotten to tell me something.*

The caller identified himself as the owner of the facility. I was immediately alarmed. *Why would the owner be calling me?* I had never met him.

As he began to speak, I noted the anger in his voice.

He began. "I'm issuing a thirty-day eviction notice for Gary! He hit a resident last night, and I just got off the phone with the resident's family telling me they will not tolerate this behavior."

Fear gripped me immediately. I broke out in a sweat and began to pace. I was not concerned that the resident was harmed, as I would have been told that on my previous call. I worked hard in the moment to steady myself as disbelief, panic, and confusion set in. I had been riding an emotional roller coaster for eight years now, and my sensibilities were damaged from the abuse.

"Sir, I don't know what you are talking about. I literally just hung up the phone with a medical technician. I check in daily. I spent the day with Gary yesterday. He's been fine. He's had some episodes, but he's had a lot of improvement," I said with a shaken voice.

He shouted, "I don't care. I will not assume liability for him!"

I was appalled that a professional would talk to me in this manner. I did nothing wrong! I struggled to retain my composure. *I need this placement. Gary needs this placement. Transitions are very hard. He cannot endure another move after only two months!*

"Sir, you need to understand," I implored. "I have no idea what you are talking about. I talk to your staff daily. I implemented a log in your facility so we could note any triggers. I advocate, and I'm heavily involved in Gary's care. I spoke to your care manager yesterday and your med tech today, who assured me that Gary is in a good place with his behavior. The medications are working! He is sleeping the whole night."

"That's not what I heard!" he screamed. He hit a resident whose family is demanding action. He broke a piece of furniture when he arrived. I will not assume liability for him. You have thirty days to find him another placement."

I remained focused, but my nerves were raw. I steeled myself but felt my anger rising. I cautioned myself, *Calm down! You need this facility! A facility you pay $6,200 a month to care for Gary!* Thoughts raced through my head. *Gary has a medical and professional team, including hospice, looking out for his best interests. Surely, they will not allow this to happen! Why is the owner screaming at me? I don't even know this man. What have I done wrong to deserve this anger from him? Where is he getting his information?*

"Sir," I began. "Please calm down. You are upsetting me."

"What would you do?" he demanded. "If it were you? Would you assume this liability?"

Did he just ask me that question? I thought.

"Well, sir, it's a responsibility you assume when you accept dementia patients. Gary had a full assessment before you admitted him. Surely you know aggression is a behavioral symptom of dementia. Regardless, the information you are giving me is in direct conflict with the reports I received from your staff. I spoke to them barely ten minutes ago."

With his tone unchanged he shouted, "YOU are the reason for these aggressive episodes! I've had sixty-five years in this business, and when you take him offsite he cannot transition back! This is YOUR fault!"

I was in utter disbelief at this accusation. Willing myself to remain unruffled, I responded. "My fault? I caused this? Gary's always transitioned well after spending time with me. Why didn't you share this if you've known all along it was triggering his aggressive episodes?"

His tone changed. He replied, "I've seen this happen time and time again. Residents cannot handle offsite visits."

"Well," I began. "I can fix that. I just won't take him offsite anymore. It's okay if I visit him inside the facility, right?"

"Yes, of course" he answered, very condescendingly. "But I'm keeping this thirty-day notice in place. If he goes thirty days without an incident, we'll revisit this discussion. But as of now, it stays in place." He ends in a threatening voice, "One more incident, I'm sending him to a hospital psych ward!"

I thanked him and hung up the phone. I began to shake. *Did that call just happen? No, it could not have. I imagined that.* I realized how differently this call would have played out years before. I would have been a screaming banshee if someone spoke to me like that. But dementia changes you. It makes you afraid. Very afraid.

This journey dictates caution and restraint. It creates a tremendous fear of bringing a loved one home that you can no longer manage; you will deal with the devil himself just to spare your sanity. You live on the brink of a nervous breakdown.

I began to walk aimlessly around my kitchen. *No, wait,* I tell myself. *This cannot be happening. I can't handle another transition with Gary. I cannot take much more. Poor Gary. He can't handle this. He's been doing so well. He's weathered so many storms. How can the owner be so cruel? What the hell am I going to do?*

The tears of panic flowed. I was numb with utter despair. *How can he do this? Doesn't he know the trauma these transitions take on a patient? Doesn't he realize all this man has endured since 2014? What responsibility does the facility have? How the hell am I supposed to do this? Gary is just now getting better. This will set him so far back!*

Eviction notice

I reached for the phone and connected with the facilities care manager. "Lisa, I just got a call from the owner! What is going on? I am standing here in utter disbelief. Does Gary need more medication? This placement cannot be disrupted. I cannot transition him again!"

She began, "He's fine, Rose. I'd suggest 12.5 mg Seroquel at 2:30 pm. That'll take care of the early sundowning. Otherwise, he's good." I stood in disbelief by the conflicting report.

"Lisa, I just got a thirty-day eviction notice. I cannot take him outside the facility anymore!"

"Just for the time being. Rose. We'll revisit the outings in a couple months."

I stared off into the room. I felt some relief but was more confused than ever. *Why is she so calm? Why is she behaving like I won't have to move him? Does that mean that I shouldn't start looking?* I thanked her and hung up the phone. I began self-talk. *It's okay, Rose. Calm down. We've got this. Everything is okay. Just don't take him offsite. He'll be okay. He won't be evicted.*

The second call I made was to Ralph to share the news. His level of disbelief matched mine. "What are **YOU** going to do?" he asked. I chuckled to myself. *What am **I** going to do about **YOUR** father?* Even though I was fully committed to Gary, it always shocked me that I was the ONE assigned the full responsibility for his care. I was the ONE who should have all the answers. I was the ONE to do all the work. If this were my father and I were talking to my mother I would say, "Calm down, Mom. It's a lot to process. You do not have to do this alone. Together we will figure something out."

There was nothing I could do but wait it out and hope for the best. I promised myself to call the facility every day.

March – April 2022

Gary made it twelve days with no episodes of aggression. I anxiously waited for the phone to ring. I turned off my phone for two-hour periods just so I could relax.

I stopped taking Gary offsite. It was hard to go there and not take him out. I'd pick up a mocha frappe, go inside the facility, give him a hug and a kiss, and tell him I'd see him soon. I was frightened to be the cause of any disruption. I'd then cry all the way home.

On the thirteenth day after the eviction notice, I called the facility at 12:30 p.m. One of the med techs answered, and I inquired about Gary.

"He's doing wonderful," she said. "In fact, he just got done eating. He ate all his lunch, and now he's walking the halls as he usually does."

"That's great," I said. "I'm so happy to hear that."

Thirteen days and counting, I thought. I knew he was going to make the rest of the month without an aggressive episode. I just knew it! I decided to go shopping for some spring flowers to celebrate, so I gathered my things and headed for the door. Just then, the phone rang.

I reached for it, "Hello."

"Rose, it's the med tech. Gary is being sent to the ER. I think he had a seizure. He fell, and he's bleeding badly," she said with panic in her voice.

Again, fear took over, and I began to shake. I gathered my wits. "Why are you sending him to the ER? You know he's under hospice care. They should have been called. We are trying to prevent hospitalizations."

"I don't know," she said. "I didn't think to call them. He's bleeding badly."

I tried to quell my anger and frustration with her for not following protocol. I had worked hard to get hospice on board to prevent ER visits, which are traumatic for a dementia patient. Hospice could stitch his wound and bring in a portable x-ray if necessary.

When I arrived at the hospital, I was petrified to get out of the car. I felt mentally unprepared to handle another ER visit. I said to myself, *it's going to be okay, Rose. It's going to be okay. Please, Lord, help me walk into this hospital.*

I was directed to the room Gary was in. No one was with him. Hospice staff assigned to the hospital never showed up. He was stretched out on a hospital cot with a thin sheet covering him. I heard myself gasp. His face was covered with blood. Literally covered. I watched as blood from a forehead wound dripped down into his eye. *Why have they not cleaned his face?* His nose was at an odd angle, and his neck was in a brace. I could feel beads of sweat forming above my lip. I suddenly felt so cold. I started to tremble. I leaned into the wall, willing myself to gain control. *What kind of a fall did he take?*

When I felt that my legs were steady enough, I walked toward him. I put my mouth by his ear. I whispered, "Hi, sweetheart. I'm here. You are safe. I'll take care of you. How are you feeling?"

He managed to open one eye. "I'm okay," he whispered. His lucidity despite late-stage dementia surprised me. I was happy but puzzled when he responded in a normal fashion. When he had lucidity, I always questioned whether he had dementia, although I knew better.

"It's okay, babe. You're going to be okay. I'm here now. Just rest," I reassured him.

My emotions were raw, and they surfaced through tears. I felt his pain. I felt my pain. I did not know how much longer I could suffer for two! My soul ached daily with his suffering. I reached for a low stool by his cot, not trusting my legs to hold me.

The doctor walked in. My head was down. "Mrs. Jordan?"

I looked up. He stared into my eyes. His voice took on a comforting tone. "What can I get you?" he asked. "Do you need water? You do not look well."

"No," I mumbled. "I'm fine." I steeled myself for bad news.

He pulled a stool close to me and reached for my hands.

"Gary suffered a fracture in his neck."

"Huh?" I whispered.

"It's okay," he says. "It will heal naturally in four to six weeks. But he'll have to wear a neck collar." I thought, *he won't tolerate that.* He continued, "I used a butterfly bandage to seal the laceration on his forehead. I'll take another look at it, because it's oozing. He also suffered a broken nose. It will heal on its own. There is no reason to admit him. He can go home."

I tried to keep my composure. *How could a fall in a hallway cause these injuries? Gary was not a fall risk.*

I questioned the doctor, "Did he have a seizure?"

He said, "I don't think so. We didn't give him any seizure medication. We can if you want us to. We just gave him Ativan to calm him for the neck x-ray."

"No additional seizure medication," I instructed. "If he was post-seizure, he would not have been able to answer me. The medication will only add to his confusion. He will get his regular dose when he returns to the facility."

The doctor and I attempted to get Gary up and into a wheelchair, but the Ativan plus his stage of dementia made him too confused to follow commands. An ambulance transport was arranged. I phoned the facility and told them the news. They assured me they would put on a bed alarm and do fifteen-minute checks.

I then settled into the ER room. I knew from experience I had a long wait ahead of me until an ambulance was available. I asked a nurse for a wet washcloth and washed the blood off Gary as best I could. A nurse came in and dealt with the laceration on his forehead. Gary remained calm as I reassured him and told him to rest. He did not appear to be in any pain.

After nine hours in the ER, an ambulance transport arrived to take him back to the facility. I cried all the way home. I hadn't eaten all day, so I made some toast and tea. I took a tranquilizer, begged for sleep, and hid my phone. Before I fell asleep, I prayed a silent prayer. *Please, dear Lord, protect Gary. Shield him and keep him safe.*

Patient dump

"The loneliest moment in someone's life is when they are watching their whole world fall apart, and all they can do is stare blankly."

F. SCOTT FITZGERALD

April 12, 2022

At 7:30 a.m., I woke up to the phone buzzing in the drawer next to my bed. Instantly I felt alarmed. I told myself, *don't answer it! It's too early for someone to be calling. Something has happened.* It stopped ringing, but after a couple minutes, I gained courage and picked it up. I listened to the new voicemail.

It was the med technician from the facility informing me that Gary had rolled out of bed and was being sent back to the ER to get his eyelid stitched. He continued, "After talking with the facility doctor, there is just no way we are going to be able to take care of Gary. The doctor said it's best that you find another placement for him. If you have any questions, call me at the facility."

My head began spinning. Feeling faint, I sat up and steadied myself on the bed. A wave of nausea came over me. I popped a couple of Tums. *This cannot be happening!* I hit the call back button and waited patiently to be connected to the med tech.

I willed myself to stay calm. "What do you MEAN you cannot take care of Gary? Where is he going to go? I'm sure a stitched eyelid will not require hospitalization."

"He cannot come back," the med tech replied. "You might want to see if a hospice house can take him."

"What are you talking about? Gary has been doing just fine. He's not ready to die. He didn't even have a seizure. You told me yourself, just the other day, how great he was doing. I do not understand any of this!"

"I'm sorry. We can no longer meet his needs."

The safety nets the facility promised to provide Gary and I dropped us in an emergency room with no parachute. *How could this even be tolerated?* I paced my bedroom trying to convince myself I had imagined all this. I lowered myself into a rocking chair. I rocked furiously. The tears came quickly. Putting my head in my hands, I began talking to an empty room. *What the hell am I supposed to do? There is no one to help me. I have no support! I cannot bring him home! I cannot care for him. How will he survive this after all he has been through? What the hell is going on?*

After composing myself, I walked into the bathroom and splashed water on my face. I phoned the ER and was comforted by the doctor on call. He was extremely nice and reassured me that Gary was doing fine. "We needed to stitch a split eyelid," he said. "I numbed it, and Gary had no issues while I was working on him." He continued, "He also has a fractured hand, so we put a splint on it. He's resting now. He is discharged, so you can pick him up whenever you want."

I hung up the phone. *Pick him up? And take him where? How the hell do you break a hand and get a split eyelid from falling out of bed?*

Because Gary was resting, I decided to take the time to make some calls. I dialed the regional ombudsman.

"What the hell am I supposed to do?" I asked. "Can they actually do this?"

"Yes," she said. "They gave a thirty-day eviction notice. I'm looking at it." Obviously, the facility had phoned her.

"But that was for aggression! He's had no recent aggression. He's been doing so good."

She told me that evictions happen all the time and encouraged me to call the state licensing board and adult protective services at the county department of health and human services to file a formal complaint.

"But what am I going to do? I cannot bring him home."

She began, "Refuse to take him home. Tell them you cannot care for him. Do not let them pressure you! Do NOT remove him from the ER until you have a placement! You can do this, Rose!"

I hung up and made both calls she had suggested and gave them all the information they needed. I then phoned Ralph and gave him the bad news. He was concerned but made no offer to come and help. *Surely, he does not expect me to manage this situation alone.*

Emergency Room

I phoned Linda to meet me at the ER. I knew I needed emotional support. I entered the ER and found Gary lying on an ER cot in a urine-soaked pull-up and a t-shirt. I did not recognize the t-shirt as being one of his. His eyes were closed. Underneath the stitched eyelid, both eyes were bruised. The laceration above his eye from the night before was crusted with blood. His nose was swollen. In addition to the neck brace, he had a splint running from his elbow down to his fingers. I noticed it was his right arm. *How is he supposed to feed himself?* The fingers that were sticking out from the cast looked red and swollen. *Am I responsible for this? I chose this facility.*

As I surveyed the damage and did my best to keep my emotions in check, a nurse walked in. I introduced myself. I asked her if we could get him changed and into a gown.

She said, "He's set for discharge."

I replied, "He's not going anywhere. He has no place to go. I cannot take him home. The facility will not accept him back. I need time to find another facility."

She explained, "We are not equipped for long-term care. This is an emergency room."

I stood my ground. "I'm aware of that. Admit him if you must, but he is not going anywhere."

She replied, "We cannot do that. His injuries do not warrant admission. He is discharged!"

I stood firm. "I'll repeat myself. He is not going anywhere. Kindly call the facility and get a list of his medications, as he is overdue for his seizure medication, and he will soon need his Seroquel. And please get someone in here who can change him."

Another nurse came in and informed me that one of his medications was not available in the hospital pharmacy. I grabbed my purse and drove over to the facility to retrieve it. The med tech who phoned me earlier let me in. I could barely look at him. If I spoke, I would

A journey of love

explode in anger. He acted like it was just another day. He handed me the medication, and I left. I was in disbelief that only a few days ago I thought this was Gary's forever home. *What the hell did they do to my husband?*

When I arrived back at the ER, Linda and a nurse who had assumed the role of a social worker were there. The nurse explained that Gary could not stay in the ER. She continued, "He needs to be placed." I could not process. I could not think. I stared at my injured husband, vulnerable and helpless. I repeated myself in a barely audible tone, "He is not going anywhere. I need time."

My thoughts began to race in a mind that was overtaxed and overwhelmed. *This is a human being! How can he be discarded like a piece of trash? He has no clothes. All his things are in a place he can no longer return to. He cannot feed himself. How will he handle another transfer trauma? How will he even get through the night?*

"Mrs. Jordan, are you listening to me? Where do you want him to go? Rehabilitation? Skilled nursing? Memory care?"

I looked at her with eyes overflowing with tears. I found my words. "I don't know!" I felt my emotions getting the best of me. I was no longer in control. I looked over at Linda.

Linda took charge. She turned to the nurse. "Can you get a recliner in here? I'm staying the night. Rose, go home. I've got this. Go home. We will deal with all of this in the morning."

I was unable to move. I couldn't stop the tears. *I cannot do this again.* I felt sick with grief. I felt I was going to vomit. *Did I do this to Gary? Did I cause this by transitioning him to a bad place?* I raced down the hall to the restroom and began dry heaving. After I exhausted myself, I sat on the bathroom floor. *Perhaps I can hide here. No one will know where I am.* When I regained control, I returned to Gary's side.

Bending down, I whispered into his ear. "I promise you everything will be alright. I will make this alright. I need you to be strong." *How can I leave him here? What will happen to him? Sundowning is going to start soon. His other medications haven't arrived yet. Suppose he gets aggressive? Then I'll never find another facility that will accept him. Suppose he tries to get out of bed? He's not in a hospital bed yet. There are no rails. How can he be made to understand that he cannot walk around in an emergency room? It's almost dinner time. He hasn't eaten all day.* Despite my efforts, I could not stop the thoughts or calm myself. My emotions were begging to be let loose again.

Linda was at my side. She reached over, hugged me, and held me tight. "I've got this. Take your time. Steady yourself. I want you to go home. Call me when you get there. Drive safe. I've got this, Rose. Please, trust me. You need to leave. You need to leave now."

I walked over to Gary and embraced him, despite the apparatus holding him together. I held him tightly for the longest time. "It's going to be okay, sweetheart. I promise. I'll see you in the morning. Linda is here with you." *I did not believe one word of the promise I just made.*

Gary tried to open the eye that wasn't stitched. "Okay," he mumbled.

My world went blank as I entered my car. I sat trying to meditate on a sense of calm. I had a drive of over an hour ahead of me. *How does this happen in the richest country in the world? Who are we becoming as a society? Why is everyone desensitized to the pain of others?*

It was at least an hour before I was able to regain enough sensibility to start my car. I somehow found my way home.

Million-dollar question: If Gary were a baby, would he have been dumped in an ER? He was in all mental aspects a baby. He could not articulate what he needed. And he relied on someone 24/7 to take care of him.

My answer is "No." Babies are much more loveable than old men or women with dementia. They smell better. They are sweeter, and they have a future ahead of them. *We throw away people so easily in our culture, especially seniors.*

The Next Five Days

The second day in the ER I focused only on tending to Gary. I sat by his side. I bought three milkshakes, as I knew he would not eat much. I made sure he received all his medications and that they were administered correctly. I looked for signs of pain. I clocked the times between pull-up changes. Gary kept wanting to get out of bed, unable to process where he was or why he could not walk around. The hospital bed I asked for had not been delivered. It was difficult to keep his fractured neck vertical regardless of the pillows I forced behind it.

I was struggling with guilt. *Did I cause this by selecting the wrong facility? Should I have done more research? What have I done?*

Hospice phoned, "Who do you want us to call for placement?" A nurse asked the same question. Ralph called asking the same. I honestly did not know how to answer. They wanted direction from a compass that was broken. They all knew Gary's history. They all knew he had been transitioned just two short months ago. They all knew his injuries and that his medications had been adjusted for aggression. They knew his current stage of dementia. They had his insurance information. I had no more answers than they. Why was I the one who everyone expected to have answers? I was exhausted from dealing with challenges. Could no one else think? Could no one else plan? I asked his son to begin calling facilities in Vermont and in my area.

When I regained some sense of calm, I would attempt to focus. Rehabilitation? I discounted the one the nurse mentioned. They had no lockdown unit. After twenty days, Medicare would no longer pick up the tab for rehabilitation, and I'd have to move him again. Skilled nursing? I wasn't sure he would even qualify. All his injuries would self-heal, and he had no other medical needs except dementia. Plus, many nursing facilities had no lockdown unit. I did this search before; most had waiting lists. Assisted living? No, that was no longer working; it's why I transitioned him to memory care in the first place. Another memory care facility? Why would another be different? Would they accept him? He was just thrown out of one. But there were no other options. It had to be another memory care facility. I could not manage his care in my home with no support or help, especially at this stage of dementia.

Another cause for concern weighing heavily on me was the cost of this emergency room stay. I did not think Medicare would cover the expense, as he was not admitted. The expense worried me to death.

The third day in the ER began the same way. The ER did the best they could, and a hospital bed for Gary was brought in. He was kept clean and in a hospital gown. I fed him all his meals and continued to bring in milkshakes. Linda helped as best she could. I got some leads on placement, but all failed. We were entering Easter weekend, and a lot of people were already off work.

Before leaving that night, I remembered the previous administrator from assisted living who advocated strongly for Gary and me. I made some calls and found out that she was now a placement director. I left her a message to call me ASAP. I also phoned another contact who had previously advocated for Gary and me. I left him a message begging for his help.

The next morning my second contact phoned back. He put me in touch with a memory care facility that might have an opening. He said, "You know I'd help if I could. I would take Gary into my facility. I love him, but I have no beds."

I called the facility he suggested and provided the information they needed. Before leaving the ER on the fourth night, I got a call that they had an opening. However, staff could not arrange an assessment until Monday. That was three days away! I did not feel I had the stamina to pull ten-to-twelve-hour shifts for another three days. The ER could not provide the supervision and care that Gary needed. Before I left for the night, I called the CEO at the hospital and communicated how grateful I was that Gary had been allowed to stay in his ER. It never hurts to show appreciation. No one had threatened to kick us out. Yet.

Gary showed no aggression in the ER but was agitated when they changed him. I considered that a miracle, as a hospital, let alone an ER, is so frightening to a person with late-stage dementia! It's full of sounds, lights, voices, and people rushing about. But Gary held his own. I attributed that to angels and the Lord in that room. There was no other explanation.

I began feeling physically ill as I drove home that night. I rarely get sick and tried to dismiss the soreness in my throat and general malaise. I thought, *perhaps it's just because I'm over tired and stressed.* Although I was in contact with Ralph and my siblings, no one offered to come and supply a life raft. Ralph made it clear that he had a life and responsibilities, and he would not leave his family. I couldn't ask Steve for help because of his temperament. Plus, he was so uninvolved, I'd need to educate him on his father's needs, and I simply did not have the patience or strength. He also remained unvaccinated.

That night, as I tried to find sleep, something jolted me upright in bed. I heard a voice say, "I've got this." I found the phone in my hand texting Ralph. The words flowed out of me as if someone else had control of my hands. I did not care about the tone of the text. I did not care if his son hated me after he read it. I did not care, period. I needed help, and I needed it NOW. I ended the text message saying that if his dad got aggressive and was no longer placeable, he'd need to take him to his home. I was willing to pass the baton even if the runner could not make it to the finish line. I was that exhausted.

When Ralph arrived in the ER late in the afternoon on the fifth day, he was very respectful and kind to both Gary and me. I was feeling more ill than the day before, and, after we spoke, he encouraged me to go home, rest, and stay there through the weekend. Even though I did not want to leave Gary, I knew he was in good hands with his son. Once by his father's side, Ralph's empathy, love and genuine desire to help kicked in.

As I started my car, my cell phone rang. It was the placement director who had advocated for Gary and me. "I've got this, Rose. I'll be there on Tuesday to assess Gary. I will find him a new forever home," she said. She knew I had contacted a facility that had an opening but mentioned that Gary needed a stronger care manager than the one who was in charge there. I pulled out of the parking lot thanking the Lord for sending me another angel.

Five more days until placement

When I woke up Saturday morning, I knew I wasn't going anywhere. I'm not sure what illness I had, but Linda had it too. We were both hacking up our lungs and had laryngitis. We were extremely fatigued and had no appetite. She tested negative for Covid, so I assumed I did not have it. We prayed that Gary would not get sick.

I fielded calls from my bed as best I could. My voice was a step above a whisper, and I slept a good portion of the day. The placement director, after assessing Gary on Tuesday, recommended a facility. It was an hourlong drive from my home.

Ralph pulled eight-to-ten-hour shifts supervising his dad. He brought him milkshakes, fed him, and provided necessary support. While Gary slept, his son went to the facility that evicted him, packed his dad's belongings, and stored them in his rental car. He said the staff there offered no help and barely acknowledged him.

The transition to memory care was scheduled on the eleventh day of Gary's stay in the ER. The placement director offered to bring the paperwork to my home because I still was not 100 percent, but I insisted on meeting her at the facility with a mask. I could not let Gary enter his new home without inspecting it. Plus, he needed to see me. I kept my distance from him and brought Chase to cheer him up.

The environment and routines at the new facility resembled his previous assisted living facility. Plus, there was a mixture of assisted living and memory care residents. The staff located Gary in a room directly across from the nursing station. Because the director knew Gary so well, she was able to educate the staff on his medications, insurance plan, habits, history, etc. It helped a great deal. I will forever be in her debt.

Ralph moved everything into his dad's new room and organized it. He had purchased additional supplies from a list I prepared, so there was plenty on hand for Gary's care. Having the extra help made all the difference in the world. After I signed the necessary paperwork, I returned home to complete my final day of rest. Ralph spent the next day introducing himself to the staff, assisting his father with eating, and observing the new routine. I know that Gary's heart knew and appreciated his son being there. I know mine did. How different this journey would have been with the support and love of family.

Gary's final chapter

"No live organism can continue for long
to exist sanely under conditions of absolute reality."

SHIRLEY JACKSON
The Haunting of Hill House

Gary's symptoms – End Stage
2022

- He is wheelchair bound with very little speech.
- He can no longer use his feet to scoot around in his wheelchair.
- His swallowing is being affected by dementia.
- He can no longer blow his nose.
- He no longer uses the toilet.
- He needs assistance with feeding and chews slowly.
- His appetite is decreasing.
- He still enjoys the outdoors and the sun on his face.
- He likes being pushed in his wheelchair.
- He still recognizes and smiles at the sound of my dad's voice.
- He still wants hugs.
- If I put my legs into his wheelchair, he will automatically reach for my foot to massage it.
- He sleeps most of the day.
- He loves it when his massage therapist gives him a massage.
- He loves being placed in the recliner.
- He still says, "Thank you" and "I love you so very much."
- He still lights up when he sees Chase.
- He still loves his robotic dog.

- He still knows ME. My hug, my scent, my love for him.
- He still enjoys music, milkshakes, and cookies.
- He still understands some of what I tell him. I know this by yes and no responses.
- He still feels comfortable with those he sees every day.
- He still has a sense of humor. He cannot crack jokes. But he will still laugh when I say, "You are STILL a pain in my butt."

His heart knows me, and he always expresses gratitude.

Gary's final chapter

Would I do this all over again?

YES.

Caregiving taught me so much, and I have grown spiritually on this journey. My value system is intact, my love for the Lord greater, and my determination to help other dementia caregivers strong.

My self-pity turned into compassion. At the beginning, I was so focused on my wants and needs. While I was important and mattered too, the journey provided me the opportunity to share my functioning with Gary, who really needed someone. Our wedding song, "You Needed Me," resonates in my mind.

I did not know my true strength before this journey. I managed to conquer every obstacle that came my way alone (with the Lord's strength). I can forgive those who I feel deserted us and not regurgitate the anger and resentment every day and allow it to hurt me. I will not let go of the past, rather I will use the memories to make me wiser.

My interactions with facility staff strengthened my belief in the younger generation. I'd be proud to call the CNAs my daughters. They kept my husband clean, lifted him, fed him, treated him with respect, and made him smile and feel loved. They gave of themselves so unselfishly despite the minimum wage they earn. I loved how they always welcomed and embraced me with their hugs. The cleaning and laundry staff always checked on me and shared conversation, which provided some normalcy to the visit. Administrators and care managers listened to my concerns and addressed them. Hospice was invaluable. All these wonderful humans helped Gary endure his final months with dignity and provided me with a life preserver that I hung onto daily.

I have learned so much about the human heart. It's not just an organ but a true vessel of love. It is something even dementia cannot steal and destroy. Those who did not visit Gary missed the opportunity to see him governed only by a heart of love. It was miraculous to witness.

I'll be forever grateful for Gary. An unselfish man who loved me enough to do what he could to relieve my burden. He never complained.

He trusted me explicitly. His courage withstood this cruel disease and he never faltered as it robbed him of everything he knew and loved.

With the lessons I've learned, I finish the final walk with dementia—alone but very proud of myself for accepting this huge responsibility.

June 2022

The Last Standing Hug

Gary was adjusting well to the new facility. He was there for a month and a half and getting familiar with new routines, staff, and medication. Unfortunately, he was confined to a wheelchair. He was now considered a fall risk, and everyone worked hard to prevent any additional injuries while he healed. Physical therapy tried to get him steadier on his feet, but at his stage of dementia Gary did not have enough cognition to process instructions. Nor did he have the memory to retain anything he was shown.

The aides would get him out of his chair and encourage supervised walks, but he was too unsteady to do it alone. The unsteadiness was due to both dementia and the antipsychotic medications he was on.

Seroquel was still being given for his aggression and sundowning, trazodone aided in sleep, and a small dose of Depakote in the morning helped with mood. I opted to put him back on hospice, as he had five slips from his wheelchair and facility protocol sent him to the ER. Hospice would prevent these traumatic events by going out to the facility and examining him.

His aggression was greatly reduced, but there were still episodes of combativeness when he needed to be changed or dressed. This is a very common behavior with dementia. On some visits, I found him hung over in his wheelchair and not very responsive as his body tried to adjust to the increased medication. When I cried seeing him this way, I felt weak, but I read that a sign of strength is the ability to show up and be there for someone you love who is suffering.

On one visit, two aides and I were assisting him in the bathroom. It was an ordeal, as Gary's inability to follow commands and unsteadiness hindered the process. Plus, he was easily agitated when he could not perform a task alone. I comforted and reassured him as we all helped him to stand up from his chair. The rate of his decline continued to startle me, and his weight was dropping every day, even though he had a good appetite.

The chair alarm went off, and an aide quickly silenced it. Before Gary could turn toward the toilet, he reached over to me with both arms and enveloped me in a big hug. I heard a sigh from both aides as they stood back to give us space.

In that moment, the world stood still. I leaned into him, resting my head on his shoulder. I breathed in his scent and felt his arms around me for the first time in months. His legs, which he'd not stood on for months, held steadfast. Neither one of us wanted to let go. My senses felt the strength of his arms, his scent, and the warmth and love of someone I had known for forty-two years.

I looked up to see tears in each of the aides' eyes. We were all caught in a moment of time. However brief, I had my husband back for what would be my last standing hug. Within a short period of time after that, Gary was no longer able to stand or use the toilet.

July 4, 2022

Another year to add to the memory marker. It took my breath away when I thought of all that had happened in Gary's journey with dementia. With the Lord's grace, Gary and I had made it this far, and we had both found a new level of normal.

I thought initially Gary would object to the neck collar, but he wore it and the hand splint like a champ. I instructed him on how to use his feet to pedal up and down the hallways from his wheelchair. He appeared happy to be somewhat mobile. His inner peace and resolve to live and do the best he could amazed me. As I wheeled him up and down the hallway, I'd reassure him, "Babe, just do the best you can. That's all we can do. Right?"

He'd reply, "Right."

The new normal was both frightening and incredibly difficult to watch. As hard as I tried to accept what was happening, some days I felt I couldn't do another visit. My husband, once vibrant and full of life, was deteriorating in front of my eyes. The disease was stealing any semblance of his former self.

My July 4 visit with him was quite different than the previous year. Our outings were limited to my pushing him in his wheelchair along the sidewalks outside the facility or within the courtyard. He was locked in a world with little speech. But behind his blue eyes, I saw Gary. And when asked to smile, he did.

I asked Linda to share the visit with me. From the first time we spoke, I felt comfortable with her. She was so willing to help and never disappointed me. If she told me she would be there, she was. I could tell when she met Gary that she accepted him as he was and wanted to be at his side. I often found her giving him neck massages and laughing and conversing with him. It warmed my heart to see that he felt so comfortable around her. I always felt he was safe in her care, and I never hesitated to leave when she'd say, "I've got this, Rose."

I knew the day would be hard because it held so many memories. When I asked Linda to join me, she was happy to do so. We took Gary into the yard. It was a pretty day, and he still enjoyed the outdoors. I gave him a haircut and nail trim. The facility was still trying to replace the stylist who had left during the pandemic. Afterwards I stretched my legs across from him and placed them in his lap. Instinctively he grabbed my foot and began to rub it gently. I could always rely on Gary for a foot massage. Some memories and instincts never die.

When I left, I reached in for a hug. He hugged me back. I whispered, "I love you." Immediately he whispered back, "I love you too. So very much." They were the first words he had spoken that day that I could understand.

Freedom

What would Gary's eternity be like after suffering from dementia? I remembered reading something that had offered me peace. *His journey was long, but the homecoming will be amazing.*

What would my life be like? I thought about that often too. Would I remember the whole man? Or the man with pieces missing?

When would I stop thinking about those who did not support us with a call, card, or visit? Would the hurt cease after his death? Or would those hurts haunt me? I knew I had forgiven them, as I no longer regurgitated the injuries in my mind. Would the Lord replace them with others?

What would 3 a.m. feel like without a sense of dread? Would I continue to fight sleep for fear it would be disrupted by a crisis call? Would I ever be able to answer the phone without going into trauma mode?

I clocked the losses methodically as my memories tracked each year. I wondered how we got here. Life was supposed to move forward. Dementia walked us backwards. Making that transition daily was incredibly difficult.

A dementia caregiver carries the life of two. What would it feel like being responsible for only one?

Dementia gained a foothold on me like nothing I had ever experienced. The worry, anticipatory grief, the aloneness, lack of hope, sense of dread, and emotional and physical drain consumed every ounce of my being. It was a cloak that I never took off. I wore it every day and long into the night.

What would my life be like after this journey? Only ONE knew.

August 2022

I continued to walk on eggshells, waiting for the next challenge to happen. I questioned whether I was being told the truth by staff. I clearly had been given false information by the last facility. On visits, I found myself hyperalert and tense. By the time I entered my car for the ride home, I wore a headache and a sense of foreboding.

Two investigations, 1) by the Department of Health and Human Services, and 2) by the state licensing board, produced insufficient evidence of abuse or neglect in Gary's fall. As a social worker and guardian ad litem, I participated in child welfare investigations. I knew that neglect would be difficult to prove. But I was at peace with the fact that the facility that had evicted him would be more closely watched. I would never know what had happened the day of Gary's fall.

With this second transition to memory care, I was no longer concerned about Gary's room décor. And neither was he. I didn't have his TV installed, as he was never in his room except to sleep. Staff preferred he stay within eyesight, so he was usually in the TV room or close by a nurse's cart. I no longer cared if *his* bedding was on his bed. If the bedding was someone else's but clean, it was fine. The days of supplying baskets of drinks, treats, and Ensure were over. In memory care, nutrition drinks needed to be prescribed by a doctor. Drinks and treats could be carried off by other residents who wandered in and out of his room, so it was recommended not to bring them. Plus, at this stage of the disease Gary could no longer unwrap a treat or open a drink.

There were no pictures of family on his walls. He no longer recognized anyone but me. I lined his walls with pictures of Chase and other dogs. He was no longer able to speak well enough to be understood or dial a phone, so no landline was installed. I didn't purchase towels, rugs, or a shower curtain for his private bathroom. He was now bathed by hospice in the facilities spa. It was larger and easily accommodated wheelchairs. Hospice reported he loved his bath and would kick and splash his feet while bathing.

Shoes, pants, shirts, and slippers, even though labeled, were rarely returned to his room. This is common in adult care homes. If his belongings went missing when he lived in assisted living, I'd get very upset. Now my expectations were different. I was different. I focused only on his care, cleanliness, and treatment by staff. I looked for dementia sensitivity, patience, and compassion from the staff, and they delivered. I will always think fondly of the young aides who loved Gary and called him Mr. Care Bear.

These visits were so much harder than previous ones. Every visit I witnessed rapid decline. Gary was down to 145 pounds from 167, and his face was very gaunt. He still had some appetite, but because of the disease, he was no longer able to process the nutrients he needed. During the visit, he slept a great deal of the time in his wheelchair with his head hung down. I bought a neck pillow, but it disappeared. The medication calmed him, but it also took away some sparkle from his personality. It diminished his energy, created imaginary visions he'd reach out to touch, and made him less aware and more confused. The progression of the disease was also a factor that contributed to these symptoms.

Sadly, we were on his last chapter. Sometimes I accepted it and did not cry. Other days tears were my only companion on the drive home. Tears had been my constant companions for so long I'd probably be lost without them.

When I'd wake up in the darkness and stillness of my room, my mind immediately thought of Gary spending so many hours alone. The hurt for him reached into the depths of my soul, and I begged the Lord to ease the pain.

Soul of a Woman

My mind drifted to Gary's room, where I visualized him in his hospital bed. His bed was wet with urine, and it had soaked into his PJs. He was waiting for someone to come to change him, get him out of bed, and dress him. He was alone in an abyss of lost memories. He didn't even know who he was. Perhaps he recognized the room he was in. Maybe the pictures of dogs taped to his wall provided some level of comfort. Was the room cold? Was he cold? The care manager had told me months ago the thermostat that controls body temperature is hindered by dementia. Did he feel safe? Did he feel lonely?

While my mind was processing these thoughts, my soul ached for the man he once was. So handsome and always youthful in appearance. He always had a ready laugh and joke for whomever would listen. His listening ear was available through all hours of the night if need be. His parents adored him; his mom loved to say, "He's my baby." He was able to build almost anything he put his mind to, even though it wasn't his trade. He'd do anything for his family—they only needed to ask. I never heard the man say no to anyone. My soul missed him. My heart ached for him.

The pain of his knowing what the disease was doing had long passed. I was grateful for that. I couldn't help but wonder, does any of our family do as I do? Lie in their bed and think of him? Do they worry about him? Think about him at all?

This journey would have played out so much differently if the family had been more involved. They would have been there to visit when their time allowed, even if it were only one visit in the five years since diagnosis. For those that lived close by, they could have visited Gary, and he'd have been able to spend time with someone other than me. Daughters-in-law, granddaughters, brothers-in-law, nieces, and nephews would have shared their memories with him. He'd have laughed. His heart would have felt the love connection it craved. He'd have received cards from them, and I'd have taped them to the wall.

He'd have been remembered on birthdays, Father's Day, Thanksgiving, and Christmas. Cards and gifts would have surrounded him. During the early years, when he was verbal, he could have had conversations with them. It would have filled up some of his long days.

I would have shared time with them in my home. We'd have shared a meal and a glass of wine. It would have been so nice not to be alone on the visits. They would have called often and asked about us. There's nothing like hearing a human voice. They'd have shared their lives with me, so I would have been able to escape dementia land even for a little bit. I'd have felt their hugs. My granddaughter would have been brought to me, and I'd have been able to hold her instead of making a video call. I'd have propped her up on her papa's lap and told her wonderful stories about him. Gary would have reached around her for a hug. He would have had an opportunity to say goodbye to all the people he had spent a lifetime loving and supporting.

I thought of those who have lost loved ones suddenly without ever having had an opportunity to say good-bye. The family that loved Gary had lost five years of opportunity.

It was so early in the day, yet my emotions were already raw. I felt tears building. I forced them away. *Not again, Rose. Not again.* I swung my legs over my bed, and I began my day.

August 31, 2022

One woman screaming
A gentleman beating on his lunch tray
A chair alarm going off
Someone whining
I steer Gary outside
To breathe the fresh air
Attempt conversation
That disappeared years ago
Eight years. How can it be?
I can't help but wish another life
Where conversation is returned
When all I hear is laughter
When all I feel is joy
It's time to leave
I feel relief today
The visit is over
I bend down and kiss his head
He squeezes my hand
Two on this journey
One not aware
The other wanting it to end
Forgive me, Lord

Gary's final chapter

September 2022

I planned a five-day escape to Charleston with Linda. I called it an escape because that's what I felt I had to do. It wasn't simply that I wanted to get away. I wanted to escape to a dementia free zone and leave the dementia cloak behind. I longed to live without the ugliness of the disease. If only for five days. It was close enough to my home that, if need be, I could turn my car around.

Linda and I rented a beach house in Folly Beach, South Carolina. We headed out on a rainy day. The forecast called for showers on and off throughout the week. I was undeterred. *What's a few raindrops?* Inconveniences that once bothered me didn't anymore. We talked before we left about a stress-free week. Eat, drink, walk on the beach, and be merry. That was the totality of our plans.

When we arrived, we settled and grabbed something to eat. Linda chose to head back to the house, while I chose the beach. As I began my walk, the stress of the year began to melt off me. The ocean sounds were calming, and I embraced the peacefulness of the night, with the waves lapping the shore. When Gary and I lived in the ocean state, we'd walk the beach frequently, sometimes breaking into a jog. My mind included him on this walk, which I knew he'd love.

Once back at the beach house, we shared wine and girl talk. Linda shared news about her family, and I reluctantly talked about mine. After seeing my distress over their absence, she encouraged me not to share. I retreated to bed and forced my concerns for Gary out of my tired mind. *Did he miss me? Was he eating? Did the staff remember to put him in his recliner?*

Day two began with another walk, and Linda joined me. It felt good to have someone walk beside me and talk. Someone who listened to me and empathized. My soul needed that. We talked about whatever came to mind, but we both kept it light and cheery. We saw a beautiful starfish, and when Linda tried to pick it up, it scrambled out of her grasp. She gently caught it and threw it back into the sea.

Linda told a moral fable by Loren Eiseley. She explained that if starfish are left behind when the sun comes up and the tide moves out, they will die. Once, there was a woman who was throwing starfish into the sea. Observing her, another woman said, "There are thousands of starfish lining the beach. What possible difference can you make throwing a few back?" As the woman threw the next starfish back into the sea, she said, "It made a difference to that one." *I'd like to think I made a difference in Gary's journey with dementia.*

Days three through five were much the same. We talked, shared, walked, sampled wine, went sightseeing in Charleston, shopped, and dined on crab legs and shrimp. I worked very hard not to feel guilty that I was able to enjoy the sea, the food, and the wine while Gary's life was so empty.

It was soon time to leave. I felt grateful and blessed that I had received a week to relax and focus on something other than Gary. At home, while unpacking my bags, the phone rang. It was the facility. Gary had tested positive for Covid.

Gary's final chapter

I'm writing a book about you

Fall was in the air, and the facility was decked out with scarecrows, pumpkins, and plants. It gave the front of the facility a festive and homey touch. In years past, Gary and I would dress up at Halloween to greet the trick or treaters. He always loved to see the kiddos in costumes.

As I entered his room masked, I found him eating. Covid did not deter me from visiting. The previous day's fever had abated, and other than fatigue he was symptom free. He was struggling with a plastic fork, causing a lot of his food to land on the floor. Plus, his food was on a low nightstand adding to the challenge of getting food to his mouth. During a Covid outbreak, food was served on Styrofoam plates with plastic cutlery. The change in plate and utensils caused Gary stress, and he needed to work harder. I made a mental note to address this with the care manager. I would also ask to have his food served on a portable table in the room.

I greeted him. "Hi, sweetheart."

He smiled. His mind no longer knew me, so I relied on his heart to remember. His vocabulary was limited to only a few words.

I quickly gathered some napkins for his lap, transferred the food to a higher table, and handed him a milkshake I brought. Today's flavor was mocha.

He grabbed it eagerly. "Thank you," he said. I was reminded of when our nieces would come to visit Gary. He would always make them milkshakes. Gary put so much ice cream in them you could barely get the liquid through the straw.

As he ate, I straightened up his room. It helped me when I felt like I was doing something for him. I brought some bottles of mocha Frappuccino, which I knew he liked, and hung a decorated pumpkin face on his wall. It made his room look festive. I also brought a TV with me, and staff promised they would get it installed. I worried, as Gary would be confined to his room until he tested negative for Covid. I turned off the air conditioner and slid the window as wide as it would open. Sixties music was playing on his radio. I began to dance, and he laughed.

"Are you laughing at me?" I asked.

He laughed even harder.

I smiled. "Yeah, I guess I do look funny."

Gary still had a sense of humor. And gratitude. He still said *thank you* whenever I assisted him or surprised him with a gift.

After he ate, I wheeled him into the bathroom to brush his teeth. I was encouraged to see that he could still navigate a toothbrush. We spent the next hour outside the facility, and I chatted with him as if dementia hadn't stolen his mind. I phoned my dad, and Gary appeared happy to hear his voice. He and my dad had always been buddies. Afterwards I shared with Gary that I was writing a book about him.

"Who, me?" he questioned.

"Yes. I'm hoping it will help people understand this disease."

"Okay," he replied.

It surprised me when he was able to process. After so many years experiencing this insidious disease, my mind would still ask, *does he really have dementia?* As silly as it sounds, the inconsistency of the disease left me perplexed.

We returned to his room, and he was ready for a nap. I had two CNAs assist him into a recliner. First, they checked his pull-up for dryness. I cringed, as Gary was always so modest. He still flexed and tried to stop them from doing this. I said, "It's okay, babe." And Gary relaxed.

It saddened me when I noticed Gary's legs no longer served him. As the aides stood him up, his legs dragged behind. He groaned as they placed him into the recliner. Although he had lost a lot of weight, it still required two aides to lift and transfer him. One of the aides handed him his robotic dog, who started to bark. Gary laughed and kissed the dog's head.

He started to doze almost immediately. I leaned over and kissed his head.

"I love you," he whispered. "So very much." As always, he extended his arms, searching for a hug. I cradled him tightly. "Me too, sweetheart. Rest now. I'll be back in a couple days."

By the time I exited the room, he was fast asleep. The robotic dog turned and barked farewell. I made my way to my car, my heart bursting with grief.

I dialed the massage therapist I hired and notified her that he had Covid. She was undeterred. "I'll be there tomorrow. I'm vaccinated. I'll bring him a milkshake; he'll like that."

I sent a thank you up to the Lord for providing another angel.

October 2022

I called a care plan meeting with the administrator, care manager, hospice, and social worker. I had several questions.

Is Gary sleeping okay?
"Yes."

How are his teeth?
"The doctor has prescribed a mouthwash he can swish around in his mouth. It will help prevent further deterioration. It's okay if he swallows it."

Any medication changes?
"No."

Any changes in behavior or sleep patterns?
"Some days he's more agitated. We have Ativan prescribed as needed. Most days he sleeps a lot during the day. Sometimes he's restless at night. We assist him with feeding."

Does he walk at all?
"No. Not anymore. He's very unsteady on his feet."

Is he still being put in the recliner twice a day?
"Yes. He likes it a lot."

I worried about the end of life. I worried that he would suffer when he was near the end. I didn't want him to suffer, and I knew what Gary wanted. He wouldn't have wanted to live like this. I knew he wouldn't. Some days I could not stand to watch it anymore!

Despite myself, I started to cry. I tried to regain control of my emotions. I hated people to see me cry. I had a hard time recovering. The journey was so long. It was just so damm hard. I looked around the table. Everyone appeared uncomfortable. The care manager looked down at the table. She couldn't meet my eyes. She loved Gary too. The administrator handed me a box of tissues.

After what appeared to be an eternity, the hospice nurse was the first to speak. She reached for my hand. I looked up at her. "We won't let him suffer, Rose. We can give him comfort medication. Trust me. We won't let him suffer. I promise."

November 2022

When I entered the facility, I found him in the TV room. Gary was allowed back with the general population after his bout with Covid. At first, I wasn't sure it was him. He looked so old and frail. He was slumped forward in his chair. His body hung slightly to the side. I noticed his right hand shaking more than usual. His hair was groomed but not as he once wore it. His glasses were perched on an unseeing face.

I went to him and cradled his head. He leaned into me. His heart recognized my scent and my touch. *How is that possible when all else is lost?* On visits, it was painful seeing him sitting alone. Lost in his own world. Even in a room full of people he was by himself.

Years ago, Gary had always been surrounded by family and friends. He'd socialize and crack jokes with a dry sense of humor. His laughter had encouraged others to laugh at jokes that weren't always funny. He had been everyone's friend. People had felt comfortable around him. He had been so unassuming and down to earth.

I wheeled him into the dining room and got him settled in front of a plate of cut-up food. I forced back fearful thoughts of his passing as I noticed him struggling to eat. His appetite had slowed, and he looked even more gaunt. Both sides of his forehead were caved in, and the skin around his mouth was loose. I watched him chew and chew as my mind willed him to swallow. The reality of what I was witnessing made it nearly impossible for my mouth to form a smile. I forced it anyway. He smiled back. I wiped a tear away before he saw it. When I looked back at him, he was wiggling a straw at the tip of his tongue. I burst out in laughter. His eyes lit up. An acknowledgement that it worked: he made me laugh.

I found myself cradling him more that day. I needed it. I sensed he needed it too. We both realized the time was nearing when our hearts would have to say goodbye.

November 19, 2022

Gary turns 81!

None of the staff could believe Gary, their Mr. Care Bear, was turning 81. Although thin and gaunt, he had no wrinkles and still had a boyish appearance. I called the care manager a couple weeks before to get a head count of all residents and staff. I planned on ordering a big cake, decorating his room for Christmas, and making the day special.

The big day came, and I picked up the cake to feed over seventy people. I also bought candles and drinks. The cake was beautiful. Gary loved chocolate cake, and I had them put strawberry filling in between the layers. Thanksgiving was just around the corner, so I also got treats for the staff.

When I arrived in Gary's room, I noticed his tiredness. He enjoyed watching me while he sipped a milkshake. I put up a small red Christmas tree with lights and Christmas balls. I hung garland and an angel on the walls and put a red valance above his window. I also placed decorative gel decals on the windows for a festive look. I played Christmas music, making the occasion very merry. His Christmas tree replaced a lamp that was lit all the time, so I instructed staff to keep the tree lit throughout the day and night.

I had hoped my sister and brother-in-law, who were visiting, would bring my dad to celebrate the day, but they had other plans. They wanted to celebrate his birthday another day. By now, I was very used to being disappointed and did not let it spoil the day.

After lunch in the dining room, the staff made an announcement to all the residents that a special treat was planned. All the staff gathered around. The chef wheeled the cake out and brought it to us. After the candles were lit, the whole room sang in unison, "Happy Birthday to you." I noticed Gary mouthing some of the words. I fanned the candles out, and we all started clapping. I leaned into him with a birthday hug and kiss. "Happy birthday, sweetheart. I love you."

I held back tears as my heart told me it would be his last birthday.

Saying goodbye

"Life is what you celebrate. All of it. Even its end."
JOANNE HARRIS

December 7-11, 2022

On Wednesday, December 7, when I arrived at the facility, an aide greeted me at the door. She told me the care manager wanted to see me. As I entered her office, she offered me a seat.

She began. "Gary's not having a good day. I've asked hospice to come examine him."

"What's wrong?" I asked.

"He's very weak, Rose. He's just not himself."

"Okay," I responded. "Let me know what they say if they come after I leave. I'm going to start my visit with him." I found Gary in the dining room, and he looked more tired than usual. I fed him as much as he would tolerate, but clearly he was not the same man I had seen a couple days earlier. After lunch, I wheeled him around the facility and then sat with him in the front room, where soft music was playing. The administrator saw me and joined us.

"I think he's losing the battle," I said. She met my eyes. Her unspoken thoughts matched my words.

After a while, as I gathered my strength and held back tears, I wheeled him down to the end of the hallway so we could be alone. I leaned into him, and I did what I promised myself I would do when the time came. I would give him permission to leave me.

As I cradled his head, I began. "I need you to concentrate, babe, and listen to me. There's nothing here for you anymore. There are so many people waiting to see you. Your mom and dad. My brother Ray and my mom. So many friends and family you once loved. If you feel too tired to go on, just close your eyes and go to sleep my love. I am okay. Chase is okay. You took good care of us. Do you understand what I am saying?"

Clear as a bell, he whispered, "Yes."

"Okay, then," I said. As I wheeled him back, I questioned myself, *what have you done?*

A journey of love

On Thursday I canceled plans I had with friends and decided to visit Gary. His condition was unchanged. Hospice had ordered bedrest, as a small bedsore had reopened on his backside. Gary managed to drink a strawberry milkshake and some apricot nectar. Before leaving, I kissed him goodbye. He said, "thank you." His eyes held so much love. I did not know they would be the last words he spoke to me.

Just then the care manager came into the room with half a dozen aides and began giving instructions on how to care for Gary while on bedrest. While they were making him comfortable, I ran out and purchased two more milkshakes for dinner and bedtime. I asked the administrator to please purchase milkshakes in the morning for him, and I'd reimburse her. She readily agreed. "Sure, Rose, I can do that." I drove home unable to shake a feeling of dread.

On Friday morning as I was preparing to head out, the phone rang. It was hospice. "Rose," she began. "We are discontinuing all of Gary's medications."

"Huh?"

"He's not doing well, Rose."

"But won't he have a seizure? Suppose he gets better? Is that possible?"

"Sometimes, Rose, they snap out of it. But it doesn't look good. Gary is not responding. We will supervise him closely and provide whatever comfort medication we must."

I hung up the phone and sat on the edge of the bed letting my tears flow. *This cannot be*, I told myself over and over. *Why did you say that to him? He's leaving you. Am I responsible for this? Oh, dear Lord, what have I done?* When I arrived at his room a priest was exiting. He gave me a blessing and left. Inside, Gary was sleeping. No amount of prompting awakened him. I pulled the blinds open and put on the radio. Christmas carols were playing. *He'd like that*, I thought. I pushed the bed away from the wall, pulled the covers back, and crawled into bed beside him. I did not move for hours. Before I left for the night, I

Saying goodbye

phoned Steve and told him that his dad might not make the night. The care manager had phoned Ralph earlier.

Steve arrived at 3 a.m. Saturday morning. Gary was running a fever. The aides instructed him to bathe his dad's head with cool washcloths.

Throughout Saturday and Sunday, Gary's condition remained unchanged. He never regained consciousness. He did not appear to be suffering. At one point on Sunday afternoon, he opened his eyes fully while I was cradling him. We stared into each other. Gary was still there. *One last look.*

I left the facility Sunday night with a prayer. *Dear Lord, if you want me with him before he returns home to you, he'll still be with us tomorrow.*

December 12, 2022

I woke up Monday after a restless night. It was a beautiful day. The sun was shining, the sky was blue, and the temperature was in the sixties. It was very unusual for that time of year. I gathered up Chase and headed to the facility. I called Linda and she walked in shortly after me. She handed me a large coffee and a breakfast sandwich and ordered me to eat. She loved Gary very much and had been such a tremendous support to both of us. As she soothed his head with her hand, she whispered, "You know how to do this, Gare."

At 4 p.m., I was still sitting on his bed with my hand in his. Just as Steve returned to the room, I looked at Gary's hand and noticed the color changing. With tears cascading down my face, I realized what that meant. I felt the presence of family who had passed fill the room to capacity. The energy and love waiting to take him to a better place was undeniable. I had felt it twice before, with my aunt and my mother. I envisioned my brother Ray in the lead. He and Gary were such good buddies. I leaned over and kissed the side of Gary's forehead three times. I whispered, *I love you, babe.* And then he took his last breath.

After a ten-year dementia journey, he was at last free. I would take his love with me. As I felt his spirit being lifted from the room, Chase ran to the window and howled. I held my head in my hands and sobbed for the years this disease had taken from both Gary and me.

The Aftermath

My Christmas tree was beautiful that year. Gary's voice had whispered to me, *celebrate the holiday with a tree like we always did.* So, I purchased one and enjoyed decorating it. The lights took some of the darkness away from the season. A photo of Gary was taken off the facility tree and placed on mine. Sitting alone at night, I allowed my eyes to melt into the lights.

Gary requested his ashes be buried with his parents in his home state of Rhode Island. Local family members suggested that I return with his ashes and have the mass at the church he attended twenty-two years prior. This would allow them and families in surrounding areas to attend. I did not have the physical or emotional stamina to travel after a ten-year dementia journey, his death, and going through the preparations to have his body cremated. Plus, family who might have attended had been absent during the journey.

I decided I would have Gary's memorial mass in February at his church in North Carolina. This would allow me more time to process his death. Ralph agreed to attend the mass and take his dad's ashes back to Rhode Island for burial in the spring. I knew returning to Rhode Island, where Gary and I had shared so many happy times, would cause too much emotional pain.

February 2023

Gary's mass was lovely. Linda and I both did eulogies. The priest allowed our wedding song, "You Needed Me" by Anne Murray, to be played. Another irony. When I returned from Europe forty-two years prior, I needed Gary's friendship so much. And on his dementia journey, he needed me.

I was overjoyed to see a niece and her husband arrive from Pennsylvania. She handed me a beautiful bouquet of roses. The years separated us, but Gary and I both loved her. The family I expected to attend did not. This journey changed my expectations of people I love more than I ever imagined.

Many friends who were close to my heart attended the mass. They supported me through the journey and after his death. I placed Gary's cremation urn by the altar, and I surrounded it with a dozen roses and a photo of him (as I remembered him best). I had shared glimpses of our journey with the priest, who was able to give a personalized sermon about the type of man Gary was.

My heart was peaceful knowing Gary would have loved his send-off.

A year later – February 2024

I often wondered during the journey, *what will my life be like after dementia?* The truth is, I do not know. The dementia journey hasn't ended for me. I'm still haunted by memories of the illness, the suffering, the disconnect with family, and what the disease stole from us. I miss the man I knew pre dementia. I was relieved after Gary passed that he was no longer suffering. I felt most of the hard stuff was over, but the truth is, once the numbness wore off, a different type of grief settled in my bones.

I know that Gary is at peace because he has sent me many signs. His spirit walks alongside me, pushing me to make the most of my last chapter on earth. It is currently a blank slate. Gary was never the type of man that would want me to cry and mourn over him. *Live your life, enjoy yourself* are the words he'd whisper in my ear.

The biggest ache in my heart is that I continue to feel Gary left this world not knowing how much he was loved. To his last breath, I know his heart remembered all the love he had for others. He could not visit them and hear their memories of him, share a laugh, give them a hug, or say goodbye. They needed to come to him. Sharing memories after a loved one has passed does not benefit the deceased.

The dementia journey was always about Gary, but many made it about themselves, the disease, or the caregiver. Many who could have seized the opportunity to show love and support to Gary did not. It's sad that they could not focus on Gary's love for them and how they might have supported that by sharing a small bit of themselves in his time of need.

Some focused on the disease and what it was doing TO him, rather than on what it was NOT. It was not stealing his heart. The heart is so much more powerful than the mind. They missed the opportunity to see it alive and well despite the loss of all else.

As a caregiver, I often felt the target of their grief. It was much easier for them to be angry at me because of what they felt I should or should not be doing. Whether they understood my decisions or not, I needed to be respected, as I always worked in Gary's best interests.

It's so critical for caregivers to be able to discuss care and vent frustrations, hurt, and grief with others. It's not helpful when others personalize it or theorize it. Caregivers should be given grace with a listening ear, hugs, and support. It's not supportive when people judge them, deny the reality, criticize care, advise them on matters they are not fully aware of, act nonchalant about the caregiver's experience, insist it is their job, or assume book knowledge is the same as walking the walk. Caregivers are doing the very best they can with the tools they have.

My life has changed forever. I think it is safe to say that this is true for anyone who commits themselves to helping someone with dementia. Connections from my past are in a healing mode, and I'm not sure the scars on my heart will heal enough to make relationships whole again. I have no regrets in accepting the responsibility for Gary's care. I feel blessed the Lord chose me. I try daily to navigate a life that was ripped to shreds and trust in the Lord that he has good plans for me.

Martina Rutledge

"Nobody has ever measured, not even poets,
how much the heart can hold."

ZELDA FITZGERALD

Martina Rutledge

Martina is a friend of mine who was an in-home caregiver that I met online. Her mom, Irmgard, lost her battle in 2020. I had the support of a facility that gave me some respite. In-home warriors do not have that luxury. With Martina's permission below is an article that she wrote that speaks about her experience as a dementia caregiver.

Today is World Alzheimer's Day, and September is also Dementia Awareness Month (with November being Alzheimer's Awareness Month).

Although these manufactured days and months are really created for other people, they always felt incongruent to me as a caregiver, because the truth is that when you are living up close and personal with one of these diseases in your home, every day is Dementia Awareness Day.

While my mom passed six weeks ago, there was not a moment on our journey that I forgot dementia's presence in our lives, and I don't forget it now. It's not the kind of thing you forget. Ever.

In the beginning, one can have dementia and still be high functioning, but as these diseases progress, they start to touch everything.

Before it stole its way into my home, like most people, I thought Alzheimer's was dementia and that it was mostly cute little memory lapses and "Oh, look, Grandpa put his napkin in his biscuit again and is now complaining that his sandwich is dry. That guy!"

But the truth is that it's so much more, and it always ends in the same way. And that's the heartbreaking thing about dementia. Even though it is the sixth leading cause of death in the US, there is no treatment and there is no cure, only the certainty that the disease ends in death. And it's not just an old person's disease either. Early-onset forms are on the rise.

The difficult thing about dementia is that depending on the person and type (Alzheimer's is just the most well-known of a host of forms!), behaviors can vary greatly. While my mom had some short-term

A journey of love

memory issues in the beginning, her ability to reason and do things like complex math remained intact for a long time. There was a period where she could figure out percentages, but she couldn't remember what she did an hour ago.

She couldn't be left alone—not ever, because her judgment wasn't great and it wasn't safe if I didn't want her heating pork chops in the toaster or wandering off and not finding her way back.

Other people have different symptoms and behaviors. But as the disease progresses and more parts of the brain are affected, eventually there starts to be a lot of overlap—mobility issues, loss of continence, difficulty processing too much sensory input at once, ability to swallow, and ability to perform self-care (a common thread is challenges with and resistance to bathing).

And then there is anosognosia, where people lack the self-awareness to know they have a disease, which further complicates things, because they just don't understand why they need this medication or why it's not safe to drive or why they suddenly need to wear a diaper or why they can't stay or go out alone.

Can you imagine as a functioning adult having someone suddenly tell you, "No, you can't go to Starbucks alone. You need to wait until I can take you." Wouldn't it make you angry? It's no different when someone doesn't realize they're not able to function without support.

It is a hard, hard road, not just for the person with dementia, but for family caregivers too. As loved ones decline, we are faced with difficult questions like placing them in care facilities (some are caring and good, but it's always dicey, if you know about some of the abuse people suffer in others), hiring in-home care, or giving up a career or working part-time at significantly reduced income and later retirement to do it ourselves.

Did you know that family caregivers provide $470 billion (yes, you read that right—BILLION) in unpaid care each year? Our out-of-pocket costs average $10,697, often at great sacrifice to our own futures. I know I spent just about my whole 401k on care for my mom, so no retirement for me.

I will likely have to sell my childhood home to finance the bills we accrued. I tried my best to work while I cared for her and was lucky to be able to work at home doing something I loved, but my hours were very limited by the end.

There were many distractions, because, hello, 24/7 care needs. And I am in no way unique. There are people in a much direr straights, and we were lucky to have a home to sell.

And let's talk about support for care needs. Not a millionaire? Thinking about using Medicaid? It's great it's there, right? Yeah, well, not so fast. It's grossly inadequate and different everywhere because it's administered by the states, and they get to make up their own rules.

Living in Oregon, my mom qualified for about 60 hours a month of in-home care (mind you, she needed to be supervised 24/7), but it would have come out of any equity she had in a home after she died.

Living in some other state, she might not have qualified for anything at all. And even worse, social service policies are woefully unequipped to serve the needs of those with cognitive decline, because they mostly focus on physical disability and don't account for the need for supervision beyond help with a limited number of daily living activities.

I also never on our journey met a social worker who truly understood the realities of living with dementia in the home. They are full of advice but generally woefully untrained and out of touch.

People sometimes qualify for adult daycare. Again, it's not generally enough to help with any kind of significant respite.

But even if you qualify, being able to go is not for sure, because care facilities (and this is true of living facilities as well) will often kick people out, if they have any kind of behavior management issues.

My mom had Frontotemporal dementia (FTD) which comes with a lot of behavior challenges. She went to a respite facility specifically designed for individuals with dementia for about a year until she was nicely asked to leave for (gasp) exhibiting symptoms of her disease that were hard on the staff.

If it's hard on a team of 10 for an hour or two, imagine how it is for ONE family member managing it 24/7, 365 days a year with no break ever.

In fairness, they did try to work with us and move her to a sundowning program, but that had the same issue, and the end result was no respite for me and no daycare or socialization for her.

We adapted, and I didn't at all mind having her with me, but it was difficult. Really difficult. I would do it all over again because I love her, but make no mistake, it was traumatic, and it doesn't end after your loved one passes.

I put my whole life on hold for my mom and did the best I could. I barely slept for the last three years but still have guilt wondering if I'd just done this or that differently maybe things would have been better. When I am able to sleep, I have nightmares about her falling, wandering, or getting hurt.

The truth is that our systems for dealing with these diseases are half-assed at best and mostly place the burden on the caregiver to give up significant parts of their life or just say "Too bad for Dad. Guess he's on his own now!"

It is perhaps one of the saddest aspects of these diseases that services often fail when they are most needed. I didn't need respite when we were in the sweet shadowing or mild memory lapse phase, but on days when I woke up to door slamming, screaming, and being called a fat, lazy, bitch until I wanted to cry, yeah, I could have used a day, even an hour off here and there.

And don't think it's just respite care. Doctors lose interest when they see that they are no longer making any progress treating the untreatable. That sad truth is that many are just not well educated on dementia, especially the rarer forms, like my mom's was.

My experience was that doctors and medical staff did not have adequate knowledge around how to interact with an adult with dementia.

This is true of just about every Medicaid social worker I've ever met too.

And then there are the people in your life. There are some true-blue friends who check in regularly or do nice things like leaving boxes of chocolate on your doorstep because they know it's been a hard day. They are golden and become people whose kindness you will never forget. I would do anything for the people who were there for us at that level.

But for every one of those, there are several who fade away, even ones you thought cared and thought you were close to.

These diseases are isolating and change everything, including the caregiver. Though I'd give anything for a few more days, my time with my mom is over. I'm not the same person I was ten years ago or even five years ago, and I don't anticipate that changing.

This was the greatest Underworld journey of my life. There's no reset button you can hit to just make things go back to normal, either. That's true with both life in general or the people who faded away.

Strangers too are a mixed bag. There are the ones who are so amazing, you could kiss them. They smile and play along when your loved one thinks she knows them (she will think she knows everybody!), kindly offer to help when things go wrong, or just treat her with compassion, like a human being.

But then, there is also the guy who uses the public meltdown your loved one is having to cut in front of you in line at the pharmacy while an employee threatens to "call someone" (aka the police) and the woman who loudly proclaims to her friend in front of your person that she "stinks" (remember I said bathing and continence were sometimes issues?), choosing to humiliate your loved one instead of just acting like a decent human being.

And, at the same time as all of that, there are moments that you treasure, like rides into the country or the same stupid joke that made her laugh every time you pass a Jack-in-the-Box

(Her: Why is Jack in a box? Me: Because he wouldn't stay in the bag) or when you'd sing together or when you'd play your violin and she'd dance like she was 17.

Or, my favorite, when after days of crabbiness or forgetting who I was, her face would suddenly light up with recognition and she'd grab my hand to tell me she loved me and for one precious, fleeting moment she was just my mom again and I loved her, and she loved me.

And then, after a million tiny deaths, she was gone.

And that is the cruelty of these diseases. No matter how much you do, how hard you try, it is predestined from the moment your loved one is diagnosed that she will die.

Linda Fiddler

"The best and most beautiful things in the world cannot be seen or even touched. They must be felt with the heart."

HELEN KELLER

Linda Fiddler

I met Linda on an online dementia support group. Her words resonated with me. She wrote the following words with the intent to support caregivers who care for loved ones through extraordinarily difficult and unacknowledged circumstances. With her permission, they appear below.

I too heard the adage, "That we as caregivers make a choice."

No! The rest of society may look at it as a choice but it's not the choice so many counselors and family members make it out to be.

- I did not make the choice to be left in isolation.
- I did not make the choice to watch as family and friends deserted my loved one.
- I did not make the choice to hurt and suffer from this experience.
- I did not make the choice to watch my loved one suffer and die.
- I did not make the choice to suffer from the financial burden and financial consequences of being a caregiver.
- I did not make the choice of being without resource support throughout this ordeal.

This assumption that I made such a choice is ridiculous. It is sanitized of fact and understanding.

The choices I did make were:

- To adhere to my beliefs and integrity.
- To care for someone, I believe needs my care.
- To protect someone, I love and / or who is vulnerable.

- To return the same respect and dedication to the person who provided me with such respect and dedication.

My mistakes were:

- Thinking that those who benefitted from my mother's willingness to help them would have the integrity to try to help her, or at least visit her through this horrible, terrifying experience.
- My error came in expecting caregiving support from family.

I will not shoulder the onus of another person's refusal to step up to the plate, by allowing myself to be burdened by the adage, "It was a choice." I did not choose to suffer.

Information for caregivers

Sexual relations with your spouse	289
Work that needs to be done	290
Finding an assisted living or memory care home for your loved one	291
Questions to ask administrator and/or care manager	292
When you've selected a facility	294
Facility care	296
Once a loved one is in a facility, know this:	297
Miscellaneous information	300
Suggestions on managing care in your home	301
Emergency room visits	303
Hospital visits	304
Ways to help an in-home dementia caregiver	306
Ways to help a dementia caregiver whose loved one is in a facility	307
Dementia Patients Information Form	308

Information for caregivers

Sexual relations with your spouse –
A caregiver's challenge

You still love them.

But you are a caregiver now.

You are tired, worn and weary.

They reach for you.

They feel like a stranger.

You are no longer connected with your mind, body, and soul.

They don't act, smell, communicate, or behave as they once did.

You pull away.

You don't feel comfortable making love.

It's okay to say NO.

But it's always your choice.

You are a caregiver now.

Very often dementia increases libido.
There are drugs that can be given to decrease it.

Work that needs to be done

- Medicare needs to be expanded to include long-term care.
- Medicare needs to cap the costs of assisted living and memory care homes.
- Medicare needs to compensate in-home caregivers.
- Medicare needs to recognize dementia as a healthcare need.
- Medicare needs to provide respite funds for in-home caregivers.
- Each state's division of health services regulation can improve care in assisted living and memory care facilities by revising rules that govern these homes so that patients are better protected from evictions and receive care from properly trained staff.
- Medicaid needs to increase their in-home coverage.
- Dementia care specialists with extensive training are needed in facilities to head and train the team of CNA's and other staff who provide daily living assistance and interact with dementia patients.
- CNAs trained in dementia who work in adult care homes need higher compensation.
- Dementia sensitivity training for medical professionals needs to be mandated.
- Dementia sitters should be mandated in every hospital.
- Legislators need to LISTEN to the needs of millions of in-home dementia caregivers and provide necessary legislation to protect and provide for dementia patients.

Finding an assisted living or memory care home for your loved one

1. The Department of Health and Human Services in each state provides an online list of all adult care homes and a ranking for each.
2. Local Ombudsmen supervise these homes. Report infractions to them. They are knowledgeable about the home you may be considering.
3. Try to find an assisted living facility with an attached memory care unit. It will be easier when the time comes that your loved one needs to transition.
4. One level adult care homes (assisted living and memory care) with coded, locked doors are the best. Those that have a fenced courtyard are great for residents with pets and provide a safe area for your loved one to enjoy fresh air.
5. Schedule an appointment with both the facility administrator and care manager. Be prepared to interview them. A strong management team—NOT price or how pretty a facility is—indicates an elevated level of care

Never feel guilty about placing a loved one in a facility, you are providing them with additional care and support.

Placement is not abandonment.

Questions to ask administrator and/or care manager

1. Years of experience? Years of dementia training?
2. Can I have your private cell number? Can I text you?
3. How many hours of dementia sensitive training do staff receive? How many staff are permanent? How many staff are from a temporary agency? How many CNAs vs. personal care aides provide daily resident assistance?
4. How many evictions were there last year? What constitutes an eviction?
5. What behaviors determine whether dementia residents must leave.
6. Does the primary doctor at the facility prescribe antipsychotic medications for aggression? Will you work with residents or transfer them to a psych ward in a hospital for evaluation and medication?
7. How do you deal with aggression and wandering (redirection or medication)?
8. How do you help a resident establish the time of day?
9. What activities do you have specifically for dementia patients?
10. When a resident needs it, are bathroom prompts given? How often?
11. How often are residents' pull-ups changed?
12. How often do they receive showers? Can I increase them?
13. Do you transport residents back from the ER? To medical appointments?
14. How many vans do you have?
15. Do you monitor dementia patients' intake of fluids?
16. Do you provide additional aid if a dementia patient uses a cane or walker?

17. How often is laundry done? Linens changed?
18. Is smoking allowed? Where?
19. Do you take residents outside? For how long?
20. Do you assist with feeding?
21. What things will you NOT do?
22. What are the extra costs? Medication management? Is there a community fee? Cable TV/internet fee? Pull-ups provided?
23. Are pets allowed? What size? Monthly fee?
24. What constitutes a visit to the ER? Who accompanies them?
25. What is your staff to patient ratio?
26. How many doctors/nurses are offsite? How often do they visit?
27. How long is your waitlist? Is my money refunded if I pass when you call?
28. Are there team meetings to discuss patient and care plan needs? Will I be included?
29. If a loved one has a suprapubic or penal catheter, can hospice come on board to provide care and catheter changes? Are CNAs allowed to empty a urine bag?
30. Can I install a camera in the room? Landline?
31. How do you deal with sexual activity?

When you've selected a facility

1. Make a few unannounced visits. The best time to visit the facility is during meals. You can observe the quality of food, mood in the dining room, staff's attention to residents, cleanliness of residents, and what their feeding assistance looks like. Try to stagger your visits: breakfast, lunch, dinner.
2. The facility will assess your loved one before they accept them.
3. As you are exiting the building, look in the rooms of residents whose doors are open (if all the doors are closed, ask the administrator or care manager to allow you to look inside). Are they clean? Beds made? Blinds up? Odors? Floors clean? Bathroom clean?
4. Ask the Department of Health and Human Services, Division of Health Service Regulation to provide you a copy of all the rules and regulations that govern both assisted living and memory care facilities in your state. Review this document carefully so you know the rules and regulations that govern the facility in which you are placing your loved one.
5. Cost is always a factor in facility care. How will I pay for it? Most care is private pay, but there are beds for Medicaid recipients. Medicare does not cover long-term care, but long-term insurance does.
    a. Medicaid differs from state to state. An elder care attorney or a social worker who specializes in Medicaid at DHHS in your state can determine eligibility.
    b. Online dementia support sites suggest putting a dementia patient's home in a Medicaid irrevocable trust and setting up a Medicaid protected annuity.
    c. Others suggest looking into long-term Medicaid with spousal impoverishment. It allows the healthy spouse to keep their home, cars, and have monthly expenses covered.
    d. If your spouse is a veteran, check with VA to determine how they might help.

e. There are YouTube videos provided by attorney Paul Rabale, who provides nine reasons not to do Medicaid planning.

I would suggest doing your own research before facility care becomes a necessity and getting legal counsel before proceeding with any Medicaid planning decision.

Facility care

Managing the care of a loved one in a facility is hard work and can often be a full-time job. It's no magic bullet that relieves a caregiver (POA) of all responsibility. A loved one should never be abandoned in a facility. A caregiver should be in constant contact with the care manager, administrators, doctors, nurses, palliative care, hospice care, social workers, staff, specialists, physical therapy, and attend appointments outside of the facility (neurologist, dental, podiatrist, memory care specialists, other). Sometimes facilities bring in podiatrists, optometrists, and dentists. Always inquire before scheduling an appointment outside the facility.

Facility transportation is not guaranteed, so the caregiver is chauffeur to all appointments, including outings and non-emergency return trips from the hospital.

Other responsibilities include dealing with private and long-term insurance, nurse assessments from long-term insurance, providing allowances for loved ones, and other financial needs. A caregiver provides supplies (toiletries, clothes, towels, washcloths, all other) and when necessary, hires sitters and a private nurse.

Caregivers should visit and call as their time allows, arrange a landline, decorate the room, attend care plan and team meetings, and monitor a loved one's well-being when they visit.

Challenges arise all the time, including hospitalizations and illnesses inside of the facility.

Caregivers are the guardians of their loved ones, ensuring that proper care is provided by the facility.

Information for caregivers

Once a loved one is in a facility, know this:

1. Report any concerns you have to the care manager. Do not hesitate! Text rather than call so you have conversations in writing. If you are not satisfied with a response, visit the administrator.
2. Mealtimes are the best time to make observations.
3. You should report a medication infraction and suspected abuse or neglect to the local ombudsman. They will direct you if you need to notify anyone else. Even though facilities will order a loved one's medications, you can request that insurance notify you when it's been received by the facility. This will alert you to medication lapses.
4. Introduce yourself and get familiar with staff on all shifts.
5. Show your appreciation and bring goodies (vegetable platters, cookies, fruit, thank you cards, etc.) for the staff. They work extremely hard.
6. Most assisted living facilities allow small dogs. If not, consider purchasing a robotic dog or cat or a baby doll when a patient reaches moderate dementia. They often provide comfort to a patient.
7. Clothes, slippers, socks, jackets will go missing despite you marking them. Expect it and report it to the care manager. How your loved one is cared for and cleanliness of the facility (room, bath, and bed linens), is more important than missing clothes.
8. Put up a whiteboard in your loved one's room with instructions you would like to leave for staff. The whiteboard can also be used to write love notes to your loved one.
9. Consider purchasing and programming an Echo Dot with Alexa to turn music on and off throughout the day.
10. Dementia clocks that tell the time of day digitally and display if it is morning, afternoon, or evening are helpful. You can program the clock to prompt your loved one on what to do at various times throughout the day.
11. Dementia landline phones allow you to insert photos of loved ones and set up speed dial so your loved one can easily call a family member just by locating a photo and pressing a number.

12. Decorate the room nicely in assisted living. In memory care, be sparse with decorations, especially wall pictures. The pictures/photos can be thrown and used as a weapon if your loved one gets aggressive. Memory care residents are allowed to wander in and out of other residents' rooms. Personal belongings might get carried off.
13. Do not leave valuables or money in the rooms.
14. If your loved one keeps turning up the heat, you can request a lock box over the thermostat.
15. If your loved one begins to show signs of aggression, get the primary facility doctor and/or hospice on board immediately. Your loved one will be evicted if they are a threat to other residents.
16. When your loved one begins wandering into other residents' rooms while in assisted living, you will be asked to relocate them to a memory care facility. Memory care facilities allow residents to wander freely. Redirection often does not work if a loved one is in later-stage dementia. They cannot process redirection well enough.
17. The best time to visit is the weekend. This is when facilities are understaffed.
18. If needed, have force fluids entered in the care plan to prevent dehydration because dementia residents will forget to drink. Staff will monitor and ensure fluid intake. I placed a child's plastic drink thermos (with a sippy lid) that had a strap around my husband's neck when he was wheelchair bound. He always had a drink available. His lack of coordination prevented him from picking up a cup from a holder attached to his wheelchair.
19. Nutrition drinks such as Ensure must be ordered by a doctor in memory care facilities.
20. If your loved one is in a wheelchair, purchase a wheelchair cushion for comfort (nice ones are available on amazon – you can have them delivered to the facility). If your loved one is incontinent, order two cushions. When one is in the laundry, they will have a spare.

Information for caregivers

21. If wheelchair bound, put in the patients care plan to transfer to a recliner at least twice a day. This will help eliminate bed sores and will allow your loved one to relax. Hospice may supply a wheelchair that reclines.
22. Hospice and palliative care are wonderful. Receive their services as soon as you can. They will provide another set of eyes for your loved ones. Hospice is well trained in bathing and will take the necessary time to shower your loved one or will supervise a bath in the facility spa. Hospice provides equipment such as canes, walkers, and wheelchairs, as well as pull-ups, catheters, and other necessary supplies. If your loved one drops ten pounds, they can be eligible for hospice care. Hospice eliminates ER visits, as they are the first ones called. They will examine your loved one and can bring in portable X-ray machines. They can graduate your loved one out of care if their condition improves. There are hospice volunteers who will visit your loved ones between your visits. They will always advocate for your loved one if they see something amiss in their care.
23. Chairside massage therapists can be hired. Most dementia patients love massages, especially if they are wheelchair bound.
24. When transitioning to another facility, allow a couple of weeks before you visit your loved one. It provides time for them to become familiar with new routines and staff. You can call every day for daily checks and continue visits once they are settled in the facility.
25. If your loved one is a fall risk, tailor risk assessment with care manager. Residents cannot be restrained, but you can order a bed and wheelchair alarm. Hospital beds can be lowered, and crash mats can be placed alongside the bed. Ensure there is enough space around the bed, so your loved one does not become wedged between bed and wall or hit furniture.
26. A facility will persuade but cannot force someone out of bed or into an activity.

Report, report, report any concerns.

While visiting, look out for other residents.

Miscellaneous information

- A healthcare POA will not legally obligate you to finance your loved one's care, but you will be the one responsible for all their healthcare needs when they are unable to make their own decisions. Try to get a sibling or other family member to share in this responsibility. It can be a full-time job.
- You may want to seek the advice of an elder law attorney. They specialize in planning for Medicaid and estate challenges.
- Medicare does not cover long-term care. An elder care attorney can guide you with acquiring Medicaid. Also, a social worker at the Department of Health and Human Services can let you know if your loved one is eligible for Medicaid and will help you fill out an application.
- Make sure all documents, DNR (do not resuscitate), living will, advanced directives, MOLST form (medical orders for life sustaining treatment), and healthcare and durable POA are completed while your loved one still has cognition. Do not delay.
- A neuropsychologist will do tests (up to two hours) to determine the type of dementia your loved one has, stage, and establish a baseline. A loved one should be seen as soon as possible while they have the attention span for proper testing. A neuropsychologist can also provide education to caregivers and help manage care.
- A neuropsychiatrist can help with long-term psychiatric care and medications.
- There are dozens of online dementia support groups. Search for them on Facebook. You can also reach out to the Alzheimer's Organization hotline or call DHHS in your area for local dementia support groups.
- When your loved one is introduced to antipsychotic medications, talk to the doctor about introducing them slowly. It takes a while for the optimum dose to be reached.
- I found methenamine to be effective in preventing UTIs. Everyone is different. Check with your doctor or urologist if this medication is an option for your loved one.

Suggestions on managing care in your home

1. Shaving cream on tile grout will get rid of urine smells.
2. Purchase chair cushions for wheelchairs for added comfort.
3. Purchase a chair and bed alarm if you are concerned about a loved one getting up without assistance.
4. Crash mats alongside the bed are useful for those who might fall out of bed.
5. If your loved one is in a hospital bed, be wary of side rails. A person with dementia might climb over them, increasing the likelihood of injury.
6. Utilize cameras to have eyes on loved ones.
7. Secure doors so they cannot be unlocked. Place locks high on the door and out of reach.
8. Put a couple articles of your loved one's worn clothing in a bag. If they wander off, police dogs will be able to pick up their scent.
9. Loved ones in wheelchairs will benefit from chairside massages.
10. When loved ones become incontinent, using a onesie that has a back zipper over pull-up will help contain bowel movement.
11. Transferring a wheelchair-bound loved one to a recliner twice a day allows the body to rest and relax in another position.
12. Crush pills in applesauce or pudding. Always check with a physician first, as many pills should not be crushed.
13. Because a person with dementia is always cold, turning up heat before the shower will help. Use a shower wand, as many patients with dementia are afraid of the water hitting their head. Large adult wipes are useful between showers or as a substitute. Both a chair and handrail in the shower are necessary.
14. If loved ones are constantly cranking up heat, install a lock box over thermostat.

15. Palliative and hospice care are excellent. If you want them onboard, check for eligibility. They are not just for the end of life.
16. Cancel hospice if your loved one enters a hospital. Reinstate it when they are back home.
17. Search Facebook for online dementia support groups. They can provide a wealth of support and information. The Alzheimer's Organization has hotline support. Occupational therapist Teepa Snow provides videos on dementia in-home care at https://teepasnow.com/.
18. Call DHHS in your state to see if there is any agency that provides grants for caregiver respite.
19. Seek as much help and support as you can get. Never feel guilty if you need to place your loved one in a facility for additional help and support. You are not abandoning them! The more help you get, the more love you can provide them. And the healthier you will stay.

Emergency room visits

1. Make sure all paperwork, healthcare power of attorney, living will, advanced directives, DNR, MOLST form, medication and allergy lists follow the patient.
2. Call the ER en route and explain loved one's history and current stage of dementia. Write down the time and name of the person you spoke to.
3. Instruct the ER desk that a catheter or an IV (if possible) be held off until you arrive. Both procedures are traumatic for a dementia patient and are not always necessary.
4. If you are not present in the ER, give instructions for a nurse or doctor to phone you before any procedure.
5. Report all infractions in the ER to the CEO. It helps protect the next patient.

ER visits are traumatic for a dementia patient.

Try to eliminate any unnecessary procedures until you arrive.

Hospice can eliminate ER visits.

Discontinue hospice if your loved one is admitted into a hospital.

Hospital visits

1. A caregiver, family member, POA, hired sitter, or nurse advocate should stay with a dementia patient to supervise overall care, assist with feeding, advocate, communicate for the patient, and help keep patient calm.
2. A living will, advanced directives, MOLST form, and DNR should always accompany a loved one.
3. Music will often help calm the patient. Provide it on a phone, radio, or TV. Inform the hospital staff of what helps keep your loved one calm.
4. Make sure POA's name and phone number are on the whiteboard in the patient's room.
5. Try to get a loved one placed in front of the nurse's station. Let them know it's important to eliminate as much outside noise as possible, and lower room lights at night. A loved one will get frightened if a stranger comes in to take vitals. Make sure all staff are aware of your loved one's stage of dementia and the need for dementia sensitivity.
6. Discuss with the doctor the use of trazodone or other sleeping aid if the patient is not already receiving one.
7. Inform a nurse to call you prior to tests, catheters, or IVs unless it is a medical emergency.
8. Review with the charge nurse the patient's daily routines. For example, how do they take their medication? With a glass or a drink straw? Crushed? A hospital pharmacy might not have the medication dose your loved one is accustomed to. Instead of one pill, several may be given. Any change of routine is difficult for a dementia patient to process.
9. If the patient has a robotic companion (cat or dog) or baby doll, bring them.

Information for caregivers

---

10. Do not assume anything regarding your loved one's care. Put everything into their care plan. For example: a) Patient gets cold. Provide extra blankets. B) Provide shower with a shower wand, patient is afraid of water hitting head. C) Do not provide mouthwash. Provide a glass of water to rinse the mouth, as they might drink mouthwash. Do not assume CNAs or hospital staff have dementia training!

11. Admission into a hospital will trigger confusion, distress, and delirium in a dementia patient. It will also contribute to a reduced ability to go home because of an increased decline in functioning. Try to get them home or transferred back to a facility as quickly as possible.

12. Review the discharge orders before the hospital returns them to a facility. Make sure all medication changes are entered and health services and/or physical therapy have been ordered.

13. Ask the hospital staff to provide a bracelet for your loved one. Note stage of dementia, POA's name and phone number, medications, and allergies. If your loved one goes for any medical test a technician will ask these questions, and your loved one will not be able to respond appropriately.

14. If the facility cannot pick up your loved one from the hospital, the hospital will arrange an ambulance to transport them back. Your loved one will be billed upward of $800 for non-emergency transport. Medicare will not pick up this charge.

Report all hospital infractions to the CEO.
Change will not be made unless people report.

Ways to help an in-home dementia caregiver

1. Offer to pick up groceries.
2. Sit with their loved ones while they attend an appointment, run an errand, or take a walk.
3. Surprise them with a home cooked meal.
4. Decorate their house for the holidays.
5. Visit with them for lively conversation.
6. Bring a DVR and share a movie with them.
7. Listen and allow them to vent.
8. Obtain information about community grants that provide respite and financial support.
9. Offer to do their laundry or clean their home.
10. Remember them on holidays as they are often alone.
11. Stop by on their birthday. It lets them know you care.
12. Go to the pharmacy to pick up prescriptions.
13. During their loved one's hospitalization, provide emotional support and make the offer to hospital sit.
14. Offer to watch their pet if they are away for extended periods of time.
15. Ask them what would be helpful.
16. Be a friend.
17. If needed, get information about local facilities. Join them when they visit the facility and provide emotional support and another set of eyes.

Ways to help a dementia caregiver whose loved one is in a facility

1. Provide emotional support.
2. Be a friend.
3. Share facility visits so they can take a day off.
4. Bring over a DVR and watch a movie together.
5. Listen and allow them to vent.
6. Remember them on holidays as they are often alone.
7. Stop by on their birthday. It lets them know you care.
8. Provide check in calls to see how they are, how loved one is, and ask if they need anything.
9. During their loved one's hospitalization, provide emotional support and make an offer to hospital sit.
10. Offer to watch their pet if they are away for extended periods of time.
11. Ask them what would be helpful.
12. Visit for lively conversation.
13. Spend the day with them shopping, dining, going to a movie or event. Help them escape the dementia journey.

Dementia Patients Information Form

Provide this information to an intake nurse during hospitalizations.

Name: _____

Stage of dementia: _____

Name of person who should be called: _____

Phone number of person who should be called: _____

TASK	GOOD/FAIR/NONE	COMMENTS
Shower		
Shave		
Brush teeth		*Rinse with Water or mouthwash?*
Dress		
Dentures		
Glasses/contacts		
Walk		*Alone/Walker/Cane*
Medication		*With glass of water, water with straw. Crushed into pudding or applesauce?*
Wander at night		*Occasionally or all the time Is a sitter required?*
Meals		*Alone or assisted. Do they eat with fork/spoon/knife? Should food be cut up?*
What calms patient down?		
Prefer to listen to: TV/music/nothing		
Miscellaneous		*Any medications you do not want used? Haldol? Ativan? Other?*

Acknowledgements

Editor: Christina Larocco
Thank you, Christina, for your great eye, invaluable comments, and attention to detail. You're the best!

First edition book and cover layouts by Maggie Powell Designs
Thank you, Maggie, for your wonderful input, answers to all my questions, your patience and getting this book to print.

Cover image: Leea Gorell, Asheville Headshots
Thank you Leea for capturing exactly what I wanted for a cover photo.

I'm blessed to know you all.

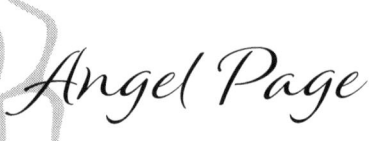

Angel Page

My heartfelt thanks goes to...

Online dementia support groups. The caregivers on these pages toil every day caring for their loved ones. Together we share our hearts, our hurts, and our experiences so that we can help each other. Special thanks to Martina who provided unlimited support, valuable information, and her beautiful article included in this book.

Administrators (notably Sarah & Joe), care managers, and CNAs (notably Tina & Jessica), and many others at Gary's facilities who loved, cared for, and advocated for us. You know who you are. I'll be forever grateful.

My therapist provided unlimited dementia knowledge and support.

The NP in the ER who shared her dinner with me.

Palliative care and hospice.

My out-of-state friends, Angela, Evie, Val, Teresa, and Aunt Liz for unlimited phone support. Hearing a human voice at the other end of the phone means so much.

Fran. Hands down, the best listening ear and dog sitter.

Melinda. A year of unlimited hands-on support and love. She crossed the finish line with me.

For all the other angels sent to me, you know who you are.

Most of my thanks go to the Lord,
who *never* left the room.

I encourage you to send this book
to a US senator or representative
in your state.

Members of Congress need to know
what caregivers experience
so that changes to Medicare coverage
and other systems can be made.

Our Wedding

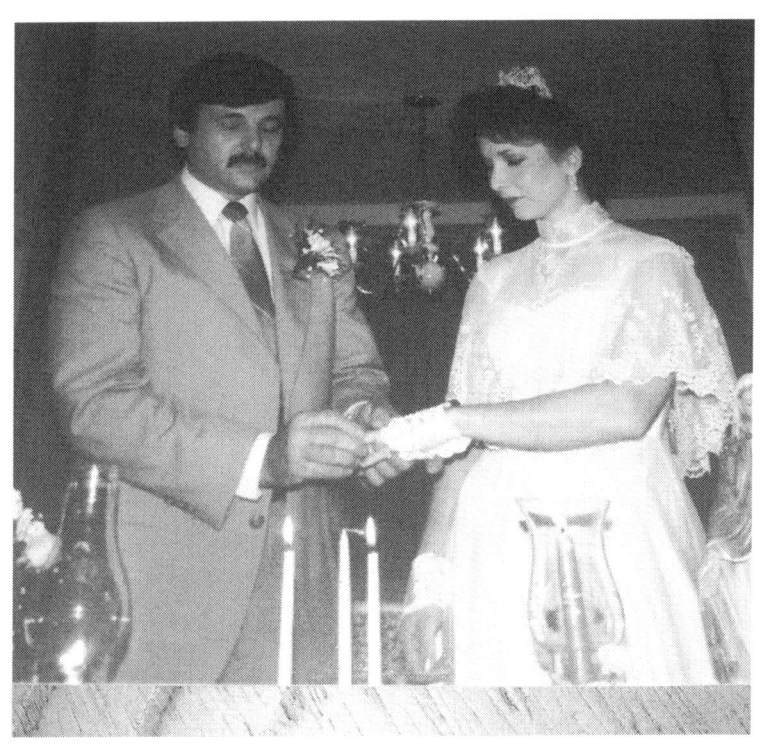

Our Last Vacation

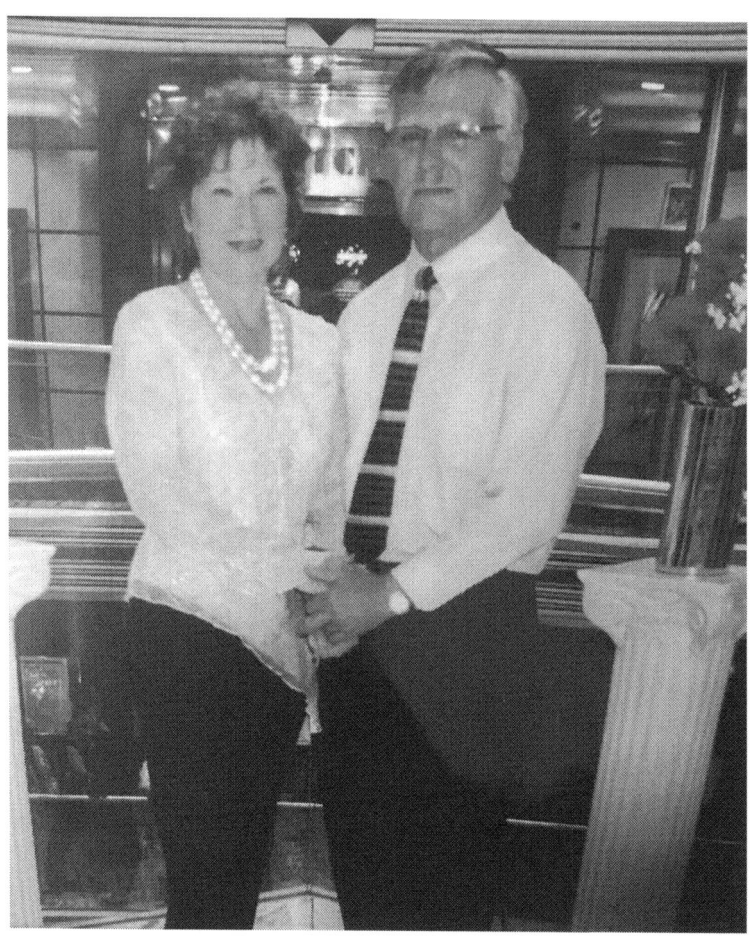

Gary as I remember him best

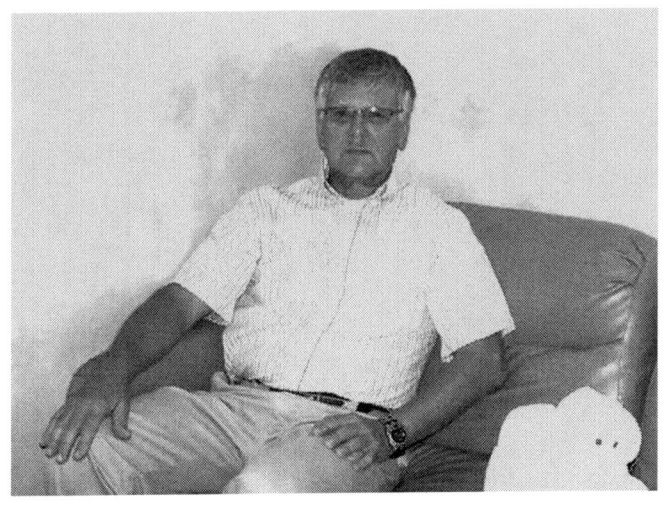

Chase

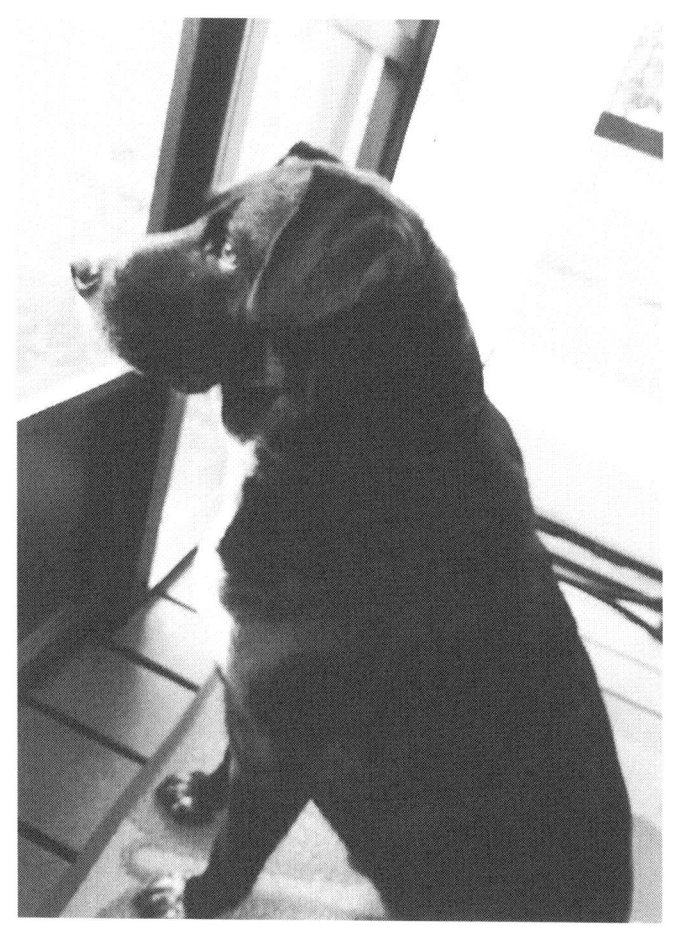

Gary and his robotic dog

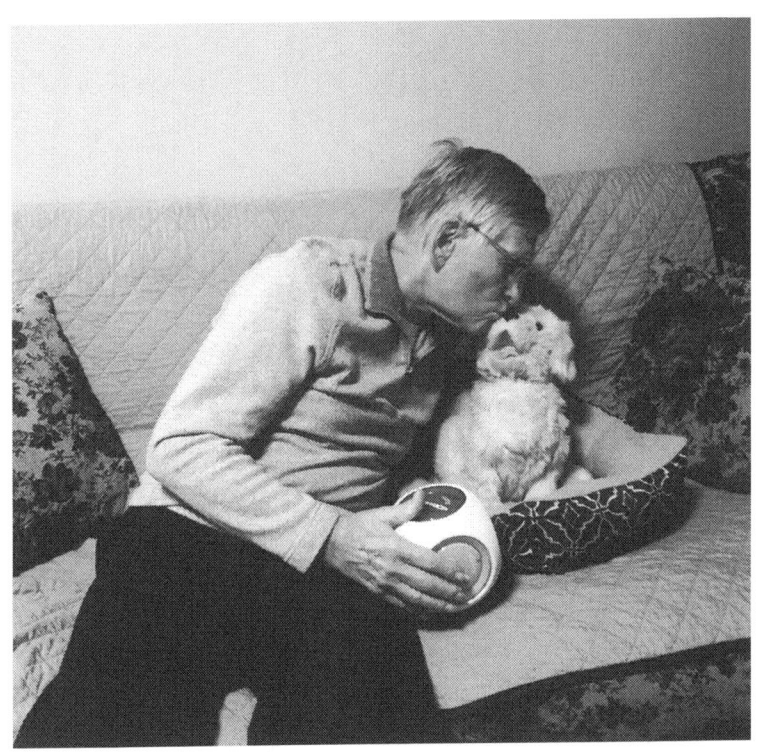

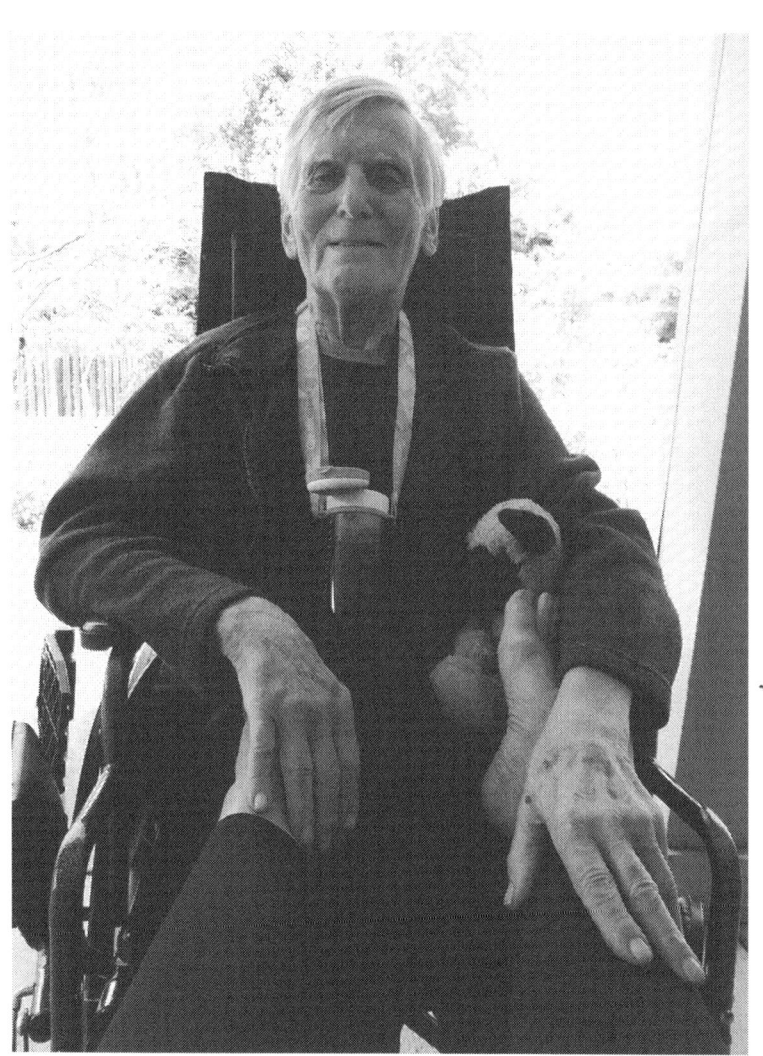

Made in United States
Orlando, FL
28 June 2025